Patient Testimonies of Psychodynamic Psychotherapy

In this unique and candid book, nearly forty patients offer straightforward, personal testimonies of their experiences in psychodynamic psychotherapy.

Both remarkable and novel in its approach, *Patient Testimonies of Psychodynamic Psychotherapy* sees experienced psychoanalyst Mark Kinet give patients the space to speak for themselves. Each case study includes a first-person account of the patient's experience, allowing them to explore what they felt worked, and what did not, in each individual case. Bookended by a thorough introduction and conclusion outlining the approaches and outcomes of each case, the book allows the reader to explore methods with patients experiencing wide-ranging psychic difficulties, from trauma and addiction to anxiety and depression.

This book offers psychoanalysts, psychotherapists and psychiatrists a rare opportunity to glimpse inside the minds of patients and explore the psychotherapeutic journey from an entirely new perspective.

Mark Kinet is a psychiatrist, psychotherapist and psychoanalyst based in Belgium. He is the author of *The Spirit of the Drive in Neuropsychoanalysis* (2023), *Psychoanalytic Principles in Psychiatric Practice: A Remedy by Truth* (2024) and *Psychoanalytic Psychotherapy in Psychiatric Practice: Premises and Clinical Portraits* (2025).

'These raw accounts of becoming mentally ill and being treated by psychotherapy provide unique insights into the real causes of mental illness (not 'chemical imbalances') and into the hard psychological work that is required to achieve real recovery (not quick fixes). The first-person testimonials are bookended by unusually lucid third-person explanations of the psychoanalytic theories and techniques illustrated in the reports themselves.'

Mark Solms, PhD, neuropsychologist, psychoanalyst and author, Professor at the University of Cape Town, South Africa

'This new book by Mark Kinet is a unique account from the patient's perspective as an expert by experience. What does it feel like for various patients to be in psychoanalytic therapy? In the commentary, Kinet, with his extensive clinical background, clearly and accessibly explains the different psychoanalytic approaches. This is practice-based psychoanalysis at its finest.'

Jos Dirkx, MD, psychiatrist and psychoanalyst NvPA and IPA, and current chief editor of *Tijdschrift voor Psychoanalyse*, the Netherlands

'The testimonies of the patients in this book are rich and varied in their articulation of the experience of their therapy trajectories, the common thread being the combination of (semi-)residential and outpatient psychotherapy, Kinet's trademark. Their honesty and courage graces them. Especially now that the – also social – importance of mental health care in general and of psychotherapy in particular is receiving more attention, the voice of the patients themselves is an important contribution to the debate. At the same time, the therapeutic power of psychoanalysis comes along in a nuanced and realistic way, transcending the stereotypical and sterile polarisation between vilification and idealisation. I believe the book will appeal to a broadly interested audience. The framing texts in kinetic style are also accessible to the layman.'

Michel Thys, PhD, psychologist, philosopher, psychoanalyst, author, and former editor-in-chief of *Tijdschrift voor Psychoanalyse*, Belgium

'Between a brilliant introduction and conclusion, in which Kinet articulates his vision of psychoanalytic therapy, he gives space to the voices that often remain confined to consulting rooms: those of the patients. Their stories are at once moving, compelling, raw, and unvarnished. When you close this book, one thought will linger: These narratives truly matter. A must-read for anyone curious about the transformative power of psychoanalytic therapy.'

Arthur Eaton, PhD, historian, philosopher, psychoanalyst and author, the Netherlands

'An original book that shows courage! Rarely does a psychiatrist give his patients the chance to describe their unique experience of psychoanalytic treatment. This is done respectfully and ethically. People who have been scarred by life early on and have carried the suffering of previous generations like a backpack describe how their therapy helped them. Kinet shows how the psychoanalytic approach provides support, inspires hope, instils insight and leads to recovery. *It works!* The reader now learns this from the patients themselves.'

Marc Hebbrecht, MD, psychiatrist, psychotherapist, psychoanalyst, president of the Belgian Society of Psychoanalysis (IPA) and author, former editor-in-chief of *Tijdschrift voor Psychoanalyse*, Belgium

'This is a very original book about the reality of psychoanalytically inspired psychotherapy. It also gives the reader a very illuminating insight into this world. This book concerns the more classic face-to-face psychotherapy and the institutional form of residential (group-) psychotherapy. The originality: Mark Kinet has dared to ask many of his patients (in both forms of 'clinical' therapies, performed or supervised by him) to write down their reflections on their experiences. Between Kinet's general but elucidating commentaries, these testimonies form the book's core. As a result, a very true picture has emerged of what this psychotherapy does to people. It shows that suffering is not magically removed, that symptoms do not simply disappear during the psychoanalytic process, but that the patient feels healed by the authentic relationship with the therapist(s), by the recognition and understanding of their suffering and by the grip they get on their life history. Truth heals.'

Jozef Corveleyn, PhD, clinical psychologist, psychoanalyst, author, and Emeritus Professor at KU Leuven, Belgium

'A psychoanalytic practice illustrates the power of words when someone is listening. Psychoanalytic authors illustrate the frustration of professional listeners – they themselves want to have their say. This book combines both. Kinet lets people tell about their psychoanalytic journey and frames the stories in his reading of psychoanalytic grandmasters. It has turned out to be a successful marriage.'

Paul Verhaeghe, PhD, clinical psychologist, psychoanalyst, author, and Emeritus Professor at the University of Ghent, Belgium

'Want to know what psychotherapy, particularly psychoanalytic therapy, entails and can do for someone? Then Mark Kinet's latest book is highly recommended. In it, he lets patients tell how they experienced their psychotherapeutic process, while as a psychiatrist he frames their stories in general terms. Not that the efficacy of psychotherapy is scientifically controversial today, but nothing works more convincingly than patients' voices. And as the book title suggests, their candid testimonies show that patients feel helped by therapy. Convincing!'

Ann Swerts, *Knack Bodytalk* (Belgian magazine, November 2021)

'The book is an interesting and complementary perspective to make the work of psychoanalytic processes more insightful, better understood and possibly evaluated. I definitely recommend it to both the novice and the more experienced therapist. The fact that all patients were given free space to reflect on their experience is a great merit of this book. [...] The kaleidoscopic perspective of the book is rich, does justice to the subjective nature of the analytic process and is in line with the scientificity of the precise description of individual phenomena, as Freud has done it before us.'

Kristel Bleyen, *Tijdschrift voor Psychoanalyse* (January 2023)

Patient Testimonies of Psychodynamic Psychotherapy

Reported and Recorded

Mark Kinet

Routledge
Taylor & Francis Group
LONDON AND NEW YORK

Designed cover image: *The Parisian*, oil on panel, 20 × 26 cm, 2017 by Steven Peters Caraballo.

First published 2026
by Routledge
4 Park Square, Milton Park, Abingdon, Oxon OX14 4RN

and by Routledge
605 Third Avenue, New York, NY 10158

Routledge is an imprint of the Taylor & Francis Group, an informa business

British Library Cataloguing-in-Publication Data
A catalogue record for this book is available from the British Library

ISBN: 978-1-032-86549-2 (hbk)
ISBN: 978-1-032-85494-6 (pbk)
ISBN: 978-1-003-52806-7 (ebk)

DOI: 10.4324/9781003528067

Typeset in Times New Roman
by Taylor & Francis Books

Contents

Figures

Chapter 1

Prelude

The Parisian

(Ekphrastic poem for the painting on the cover by Steven Peters Caraballo)

Are you looking at your feet, or are you
Looking inwards? Your countenance,
Subdued. Your posture,
Silence and repentance.

Your body is lacking. So are your hands. At most, you show the halting
Hollow of your head. And *What are you doing in Paris?*

You are still young and unwrinkled.
Your beard, however, shows an age,
Suspect.

Is it a mask, or is it
An incredibly detailed imprint of
An expression that expires

Precisely at the moment when
You borrow your shoulder
For some cross?

Mark Kinet

DOI: 10.4324/9781003528067-1

Chapter 2

Setting the Stage

I Design

This book is the third in my trilogy on psychodynamic psychiatry at Routledge. Like the previous ones, it is based on an English translation and adaptation of a book published in Dutch in the *Psychoanalytisch Actueel* (Current Psychoanalytics) series. In the first volume, I outlined several underlying inspirations for my (clinical) psychotherapeutic activities. A wide range of psychoanalytic perspectives were reviewed. In the second, I presented seventy-seven patients. I used a cross between biography and radiography. The psyche is invisible, but I made it somewhat visible. This third book is different, but it also complements the previous two. On the one hand, it consists of an introduction and conclusion with my general contextual commentary. The tone is narrative, and I omit the references or notes that were abundant in my first book. Above all, in the main part of this book I let thirty-eight patients have their say here. This time, they tell, in their own words, how they experienced their psychotherapeutic process. In psychoanalytic annals, much can be read about patients and their treatment. However, we very rarely hear their voices. This book provides an answer to this lacuna and is, therefore, something of an anomaly.

For the Dutch version, I contacted seventy patients, asking them each to write a truthful account within approximately 2,500 words. The reader can find copies of my invitation in the *Modus Operandi*, a section at the back of this book that outlines the process and guidelines for patient contributions. I was their treating psychiatrist and either also took care of psychotherapy myself and/or provided process guidance during or after clinical psychotherapy. Since process guidance is an invention of my own, I must explain it briefly. As a psychoanalytically trained psychiatrist, I cannot personally take on all patients for psychotherapy. However, individual and group process guidance allows me, in consultation with the patient and psychotherapist, to monitor, facilitate and, where possible, catalyse the progress of the therapeutic work.

Ultimately, thirty-one patients responded to my request for reports. This met my prior estimate when I budgeted an acceptable volume for the publication. I

DOI: 10.4324/9781003528067-2

assumed the task I set them for would be a serious confrontation. Undertaking it within a limited timeframe and space is also far from easy. Every bird sings as it is beaked, and, according to the Count de Buffon, style is the person themselves. Therefore, I limited myself to linguistic editing. The majority of the witnesses underwent a period of clinical psychotherapy: 24-hour and/or day treatment. All of them also had a long period of outpatient psychoanalytic psychotherapy. A minority were only in outpatient psychotherapy, on the couch or face-to-face. Following this English version, I contacted a further ten patients. This time, seven of them wrote a testimony, bringing the total in this book to thirty-eight.

2 Beyond the Wellness Spa

Except for a few individuals here and there, they initially did not ask for psychotherapy and even less for psychoanalysis. They had various complaints or problems and wanted to feel better – preferably as quickly as possible. However, the psychiatric hospital is not a *wellness spa*, where the client is expected to be able to leave with a 'good feeling'. Borrowing from the famous *Hand Oracle* of Spanish Jesuit and cynic Baltasar Gracian, it requires just as much learning to do nothing as to do something. Shouldn't we first build trust and try as best as possible to understand what is wrong or what is amiss? What is the point of a superficial or cosmetic approach when, at a deeper level, dark forces continue to proliferate? For example, some phenomena are often repeated throughout the patient's life. Where and when should we look for the roots of this weed so that they do not keep reappearing – often to the point of annoyance or – as if from nowhere?

We have all learned to drive in a certain way at some point. A breakdown or an accident can happen to anyone, but when we repeatedly have technical problems, go off the road, crash into a tree, receive fines for traffic offences, or collide with other road users, there is more to it. A visit to the *car wash* will do little good. Instead, we should subject our vehicle or driving style to closer examination. In all probability, hidden defects underlie the recurring difficulties. Unless we expose and address this problem at its root, a sufficiently lasting solution to the problem will likely remain elusive.

3 A Naturalistic Approach

Based on scientific research, the efficacy of psychotherapy is now undisputed. Different treatment forms have equivalent effects on disease signs and symptoms. In the psychotherapy world, this was long called the Dodo bird verdict, after a passage from Lewis Carroll's *Alice in Wonderland*: everyone has won and must receive a prize. It was attributed to a common ground shared by all forms of psychotherapy, which are then called non-specific therapeutic factors. Thus, almost half of the psychotherapeutic effect would have to do with support, the quality of the therapeutic relationship, empathy and 'belief' in the therapist/therapy. These 'big four' are heavily weighted and effective regardless of the theoretical model used by the therapist.

However, the aforementioned (as well as pharmacotherapeutic) effect research is often far removed from concrete clinical practice. From academic research, cohorts of purified patients are compiled. They are treated straight-forwardly, according to protocols and compared with a similarly simply trea-ted (or placebo-treated) control group. In other words, it is an artificial treatment design. Matters are presented straightforwardly, which fundamen-tally differs from how things are in real life. This book fits more into the fra-mework of naturalistic research. It studies practice *as it is*. It is often characterised by both diagnostic and (psycho)therapeutic complexity.

4 The Inevitable Detour

Psychoanalysis does not try to reduce this complexity but rather to express it and allow it to come into its own. I can illustrate this with the following dia-gram from the clinic. It describes the shortest route between two points: in the natural sciences and the humanities.

When I posted this drawing on social media, I received many confirming responses from colleagues in mental health care. It is recognisable clinically. In practice, the shortest way is indeed invariably a detour. People go to great lengths when it comes to exploring their emotional life. When they encounter painful points, they turn back or suddenly head off in an unexpected direction. Then

Natural Sciences:

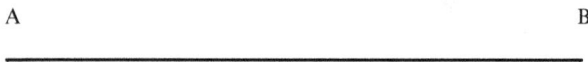

Humanities:

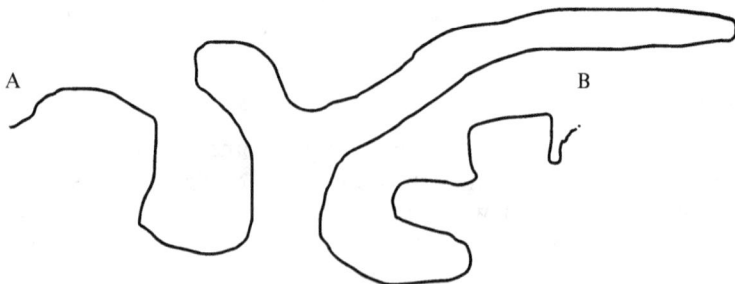

Figure 2.1 The inevitable detour.

again, they take flight forward and shoot past their target. All this is not only a disadvantage. A huge plus of such a detour is that it opens up illuminating perspectives on the landscapes of their minds that would otherwise wholly escape their field of vision.

The same drawing can also illustrate the difference between a natural sciences logic and a humanities logic. We inhabit three worlds: the world of dead matter or the lithosphere, living beings or the biosphere, and the world of the spirit or the noosphere. These spheres emerge from each other: one is a necessary but insufficient condition for the next. Humans are subject to physical and biological laws, but, in addition to these universal laws, specifically human regularities are often only effective – in an irreducibly particular way – in the head and the heart of this one patient. They depend on those specific space- and time-bound circumstances within which they occur and where they acquire their meaning. They only apply – and can, in other words, only be understood – within their specific context.

The fact that the Earth revolves around the sun is explained by gravity. The fact that the moth revolves around the lamp is explained less linearly by its need for light. Why humans beat around the bush cannot be derived or understood from physical forces or biological needs. Only the complex interplay of forces and meanings determining their mental life is responsible for these circular movements. Therefore, another word about major and minor causes and how severe mental suffering is. A stone thrown into a pond gives large waves, a pebble gives only small ripples. In mental matters, however, not only the size or weight but also the *meaning* of the projectile determines its impact. Regarding the severity of psychological or psychiatric problems, patients often measure their difficulties or trajectories against those of others. However, the cross *you* must bear is invariably weighing the heaviest. We each also go our own way.

5 The Therapeutic Relationship

It is generally accepted that the effectiveness of any psychotherapy largely depends on the quality of the therapeutic relationship. It is the main non-specific or generic factor and a necessary but insufficient condition. It concerns attunement, understanding, empathy, predictability, reliability, positive acceptance and other elements that determine good (enough) parenting. Psychoanalysis developed numerous names and concepts for this domain, precisely like the Inuit, who are said to have many words for snow. The therapeutic relationship is the basis and bearer of the entire psychotherapeutic undertaking. Building a bond with a wide variety of patients and maintaining and developing this bond on good and bad days is not self-evident. Paradoxically, psychoanalytic thought makes a particular contribution to this non-specific task.

A coherent, meaning-giving theory is also necessary to guide the psychotherapeutic process. In a witty remark by the Dutch author Arnon

Grunberg, it is no longer the priests but the therapists who give meaning to suffering. Today's four university-recognised schools of thought are behavioural therapy, systemic therapy, experiential psychotherapy and psychoanalytic psychotherapy. According to Freud, only those who use the specific concepts of transference and resistance may call their practice psychoanalytic.

6 The Psychoanalytic Approach

Unlike, for example, more medical and/or symptom- or solution-oriented approaches, the psychoanalytic approach does have its specificity. First, its intensity. The patient came five to six times a week to the classical cure. This frequency was necessary so the psyche could unfold profoundly and in detail. This frequency is rarely used today. Three to five weekly sessions remain the gold standard within the training framework to become a psychoanalyst. On the other hand, a minimum frequency remains vital to this day. This often involves one or two outpatient sessions and three or more per week (semi-) residential. If there is insufficient regularity, the patient's speech risks being limited to the latest news. Getting to the point then becomes problematic. Moreover, the thread must be picked up each time and can be more challenging to unravel.

The patient is asked to lie horizontally on the couch in the classic setting. They let themselves sink, assuming a peculiar position distinguishing psychoanalytic speech from everyday speech. All the more so, since the analyst sits behind the couch and out of the patient's field of vision. Visual stimuli or reactions are thus reduced to a minimum. There is nothing to see. Infrastructurally, priority is also given to speaking and listening to words. To their meanings and the emotional charge they contain, as revealed, for example, in volume, tone, rhythm or melody. Equally, one listens to the silences, what is not said, when, and why.

The aim of this set-up is that the patient should, as it were, be able to let themselves go. They exchange their focus on external reality for that on internal reality. They even turn away from reality to some extent and make (more) room for their mental or even fantasy life. As described in this book, the epitome of the practice is, however, equally psychoanalytic *play* therapy. Here, the therapist must leave their armchair and go down to the floor to engage with words and images or play together to participate in the encounter, guard boundaries and maintain a reflective mode.

The mouth overflows with what the heart is filled with. It is *the* working principle of free association. This fundamental rule is the characteristic of the psychoanalytic undertaking. James Strachey (editor and translator of the *Standard Edition* of Freud's collected works) calls free association the primary instrument for a scientific investigation of the human mind. By free-associating, the patient lets go of their rational control. The connections are no longer logical but associative. We believe we are masters in our own house, but it turns out that 'it' also speaks or haunts within us. This free association is more of a rule than an invitation. A certain psychoanalytic kind of work is required of the patient. They are expected to try to say everything that comes to mind and what is happening within them without a filter. The intention is that they talk past their mouth. That they say more or different things than they would like to say. In this way, sooner or later, things are brought up that are not told anywhere else: not to parents or family, not to a partner, not to best friends and not even to themselves. In this way, all kinds of unspoken thoughts, feelings and fantasies can see the light of day and often change in appearance simply because of that. In this regard, I like to quote the Dadaïste poet Tristan Tzara: *La pensée se fait dans la bouche.* Thought is (I would add 'only') formed in the mouth.

It is not just work here, but hard labour, consciously alluding to the delivery room, because all this does not happen automatically. The word 'free' in free association is paradoxical. For in the first instance, it is not free at all. All kinds of resistance will hinder the patient in fulfilling the requested task. Psycho-analysis does not remove these resistances. Instead, it derives its particular effectiveness from exposing the internal interplay of forces that underlie them.

For their part, the analyst cleverly plays dumb. In feigned ignorance, they suspend their knowledge to make way for the unconscious knowledge in the patient's mind. This unconscious contains the keys to what drives the patient's life and restricts their existence. Why, for example, does the patient always have trouble with authority, loss, rivalry, separation or sexuality? This is not written in the stars but in our unconscious.

A famous comparison is that the patient must act like a train passenger describing the fleeting landscape passing by the window (in this case, of their mind). The analyst, for their part, listens to the story with an evenly sus-pended and free-floating attention. Later, psychoanalytic authors try to describe or refine this unique listening attitude. Theodor Reik speaks of lis-tening with a third ear. Joseph Sandler speaks of free-floating responsiveness. Wilfred Bion speaks of a state of reverie. I prefer an expression by Thomas Ogden. He speaks of conversations at the frontier of dreaming. It is like walking along the ever-changing and erratic tidemark that separates the con-scious land and the unconscious water.

I immediately refer to that other crucial psychoanalytic peculiarity, namely its hypothesis of the unconscious. Freud was an *Enlightenment* thinker. At first glance, he tried to understand irrational phenomena such as dreams, slips of the tongue or symptoms through a hidden, underlying rationality. According to him, our unconscious contains the laws and knowledge of what is repeated. I quote Polonius from Shakespeare's Hamlet: *Though this be madness, yet there is method in 't.*

There is the dynamic unconscious, first mapped by Freud, which underlies the return of the repressed. You push and hold a ball underwater with con-siderable effort. Still, sooner or later, it pops up, after an invisible and enig-matic course, in an unexpected place and as if from nowhere. The veiled return of the repressed underlies many symptoms/surface phenomena. In addition, the automatic unconscious programs our actions outside our awareness. The basis for this lies already in our prehistory or later developments that have become automated over time – fortunately or unfortunately.

A specific psychoanalytic element is transference. We wear invisible glasses. Their lenses have the colour and distortions of our inner world and our past, causing us to see the same things or people often and consequently react to them in a stereotypical emotional or interactional way.

Another specific psychoanalytic point of attention is resistance. This refers to resistance to change (psychoanalyst and business psychologist Manfred Kets de Vries: *The only person who welcomes change is a wet baby*) and resistance to knowledge that we do not (want to) know. In the middle of our field of vision, there is a blind spot. This poor eyesight characterises, not least, our rear-view mirror, which often contains multiple blind spots. The psychotherapist is like a third party who can draw attention to what escapes our reflection. We look the other way for things we do not like seeing in others or ourselves.

Finally, the psychoanalytic approach is characterised by an – certainly not insignificant – additional aim. In a winged formulation by the former editor-in-chief of the Dutch *Tijdschrift voor Psychoanalyse,* Michel Thys, it primarily strives to become-better-by-truth. In psychoanalytic therapy, it is indeed not love but the love of truth that is most important. As a welcome spin-off, it improves things through greater self-knowledge. Treatment does not take place in a chemical, magical or technical way. The focus is on what makes our clock tick or not tick. Often, this concerns things we are unaware of, which determine our (inter)actions.

Within these broad lines, it is up to each psychoanalytic therapist to provide their answers and bear responsibility. In more contemporary terms, the psychoanalyst works through relationship and interpretation. The relationship is the matrix (literally: womb) of the psychoanalytic process. Within the therapeutic relationship, specific emotional or interactional patterns can (or rather, will) be repeated. This therapeutic relationship can offer a healing experience that can still be internalised. We not only do what we say but also say what we do. This whole event is constantly provided with subtitles and footnotes so that the patient becomes as aware as possible of this experience. That is also the aim of every interpretation: to illuminate the unconscious or to facilitate its expression.

7 Setting the Stage

I will not spoil the plot or the pleasure (at least of reading) by getting ahead of the reporters on duty. Only later will I conclude on the therapeutic assumptions or presumptions that psychoanalytic therapies make. However, I will first provide some further context. I consider it necessary to understand the patients' stories properly.

We all know the following proverb: as the clock ticks at home, it ticks nowhere else. Therefore, each of us is always different. In such a psychoanalytic approach, mental problems are often nothing more or less than enlargements of general human problems. We do not choose where our cradle stands. We are thrown into the world and try to make the best of it. It is making the best of a difficult job. We can get stuck in choices that have become ingrained in our development. Or, paraphrasing the words of the Nigerian author Ben Okri, we are born into the dreams of others; sometimes, we remain caught in them.

Reflecting on our history and reading between the lines of what is written, why and how (or not) can help to give our feelings and sensitivities their place. Healing or integrative experiences can also occur within the relationship with the psychotherapist. Psychotherapy offers a safe space to get in touch with our feelings and to express them constructively. It is a free space to play, create, invent and discover. It is also where old and recurring patterns can come alive on stage. They can be analysed and processed so that stereotypical, sterile or counterproductive mechanisms – often with much trial and error and varying success – can be broken, adjusted or made meaningful.

8 Clinical Psychotherapy

People end up 'in psychiatry' because they can no longer 'hold' themselves (well/right). They can no longer hide that something is wrong. People in out-patient psychotherapy may suffer severely mentally, but they can still manage pretty well. At least as far as their public life is concerned. Often, it is only apparent to themselves and/or their house or bedroom companions that there is a problem (or how big their problem is).

Within mental healthcare, psychotherapy can be offered in all settings, including within a psychiatric ward in a general hospital (PWGH). However, a clinical psychotherapeutic ward in a psychiatric hospital (PH) does not offer psychotherapy *in* but *uses* the clinic. The clinical environment offers safety, boundaries, support and structure in a sophisticated way. Everything happening there is interrelatedly aimed at achieving the psychotherapeutic goals. It promotes emotional growth and development and increases insight into the problems' psychogenesis and psychodynamics. It differs from the natural environment in that it is characterised by sustained attention, care and communication about emotional life. Psychotherapy, pictorial, musical and dance expression are core activities within the programme. They are pillars that are offered both in groups and individually.

Within the type of work psychotherapy, the rule of free association applies. It is psychoanalytic therapy in and not of the group. When the patient is not yet very good at talking about emotional content, images or sounds can help to express them. The therapist provides the necessary translation work. In addition, an arsenal of therapeutic encounters and activities is offered. They are designed interconnectedly and tailored to insight and development as 'work'.

The patient learns from the possibilities, difficulties, and ups and downs that this entails knowing or extending themselves and their boundaries or reach.

9 Integration: A Bio-Psycho-Social Model Revisited

Clinical psychotherapy enables an integration of psychiatry and psychotherapy. As an applied natural science, psychiatry wants to cure diseases, limit organic or functional damage, and reduce or alleviate symptoms and complaints. At the same time, it often sits uneasily astride the natural sciences and the humanities. Of all medical specialities, it is exceptionally non-veterinary. Humans are, after all, speaking beings seeking meaning and purpose. They are not one but two with nature; above this chasm, they hang somewhere between abyss and airman.

Clinical psychotherapy combines biological, social and psychological treatment, also known as pharmacotherapy, sociotherapy and psychotherapy. The origin of psychiatric difficulties is, after all, always complex and multi-factorial. A variable alloy of nature and nurture, predisposition, environmental influences and history exists. Every newborn brings a biological constitution from the outset. Especially in the early years of life, a more or less secure attachment is established. Throughout our lives, we try to make something of our history and the characters that appear in it.

The bio-psycho-social model of Georg Engel is fully applicable, with the proviso that I prefer to call it a bio-socio-psychic model and that the psychic is by no means limited to the conscious. There is always an interplay between the physical body and brain, the biological/ethological that we share with other (especially mammalian) animals, and the psychic that attempts to establish itself as a specifically human meaning-giving dimension on all this. 'Attempts' because complete mastery of the three registers is impossible. We are marked by a want-to-be that we can never fully articulate.

A confidential, collaborative relationship is a given to some patients and, for others, is a (sometimes arduous) task. For an absolute minority of patients, biological treatment plays a significant role; for most, a generally diminishing supporting role. In a metaphor I also use with the patient, medication can throw oil on the waves so they do not cause flooding or even more havoc. Meanwhile, psychotherapeutically, dykes are being built, and the patient (who often feels themself going under) learns, so to speak, both to sail and to swim. Psychoanalysis tries to make more conscious of what is unconsciously at work. In a famous statement, Freud compares this work to the reclamation of the Zuiderzee. I immediately add that there is still sufficient room for wetness on both sides of the bar.

10 The Patient

Many cultural critics believe we live in a time of care and knowledge 'companies'. It is a time when economics and management (as well as their language) dominate. What is true has become a commodity, and humans are increasingly reduced to consumers or clients. This book explicitly gives the floor to the patient. Etymologically (Latin: *patiens*), it is not about a customer but about someone who suffers – patiently or not.

At the age of seventy-four, Freud states in his book *Civilisation and Its Discontents* that suffering threatens us from three sides. From our bodies, which are destined for decay and decomposition and cannot miss pain and fear as warning signals. From the outside world, which can rage against us with omnipotent, relentless, destructive forces. And, finally, from relationships with other people. He says we experience the suffering stemming from this last source with perhaps the greatest sorrow. We regard it as an unnecessary addition, although it is as fatal and unavoidable as suffering from other sources.

Psychoanalysis, moreover, focuses not only on relationships with other people but also on ourselves. Unlike our animal brothers and sisters, humans have a dual cultural historicity that leaves its mark on these relationships: that of upbringing and that of civilisation. Both components of culture are primarily due to the renunciation of drives. Raw or crude sexual, aggressive and selfish tendencies are thereby redirected in a pro-social direction. At the same time, an inner conflict inevitably arises between such drives and prohibitions that regulate or tame them.

Borrowing from Friedrich Nietzsche, humans are sick animals for other reasons. Their minds are divided into a conscious and an unconscious department and, therefore, their lives are teeming with misunderstandings and failures. As language animals, they owe all this to human symbolic language. This language is our home, but it is also a prison from which we periodically want to escape (towards an idolised immediacy).

The Sickness Called Man (after a novel title and account of the protagonist's psychoanalysis by the Italian Ferdinando Camon) is also related to our three-part brain, which stems from our natural history. There is the brainstem, which we share with reptiles, where various physical homeostases are monitored and regulated. There is the limbic system, where our instincts and emotions reside, which we have had in common with other mammals for 250 million years. Most significantly, we differ from other animals regarding the cerebral cortex in our forehead. Both in terms of volume and number of connections, this so-called prefrontal neocortex is proportionally much more prominent in humans. It provides inhibition – in short, not doing something – and makes thinking and symbolisation possible, leading to the fact that we have become largely unaware of our fundamental driving forces.

In addition to the history of our species, our individual history also leaves its mark. The baby's brain is about a quarter the size of an adult's. Positive and stimulating environmental influences promote and negative or invalidating ones hinder its development. The brain doubles in volume in the first year of life, and by age five, it is ninety per cent adult. This has to do with ever-increasing connectivity between nerve cells. Roughly speaking, deeper structures mature earlier, and only in young adulthood do so-called higher functions, such as thinking and judgement, reach their peak. In short, the brain tissue and the tissue of stories and characters stored in it place us willy-nilly before a vessel full of contradictions.

11 An Internally Divided Being

Borrowing from Heraclitus, the character is our fate. Or Aristotle: we are what we repeatedly do. The laws and the knowledge of these repetitions are to be found in our character – and the largely hidden history that underlies it. Our past is, therefore, at work within us in two different ways. From the annual tree trunk rings, you can read which (e.g. warm or cold, dry or humid) seasons it has experienced. They are ingrained in it without the tree being able to tell them, but they exert their influence. Just as moisture problems can rise from our 'cellar' and repeatedly leave their mark on the present.

Our memory is also divided into prehistory and history. We cannot remember anything from our first years of life. We have to make do with archaeological finds and stories from other sources. Above all, their scenarios and templates eventually appear interactively on stage in the psychotherapeutic space. Thus, this (hi)story appears in a reprint, as it were, and therefore allows itself to be read. We begin to write and rewrite our history after sufficient (language and other) development. We evolve from pictorial or musical to verbal forms of expression, which we continue to edit depending on an ever-changing perspective – and, indeed, in psychotherapy. At first, perhaps to embellish them, later to get closer to the truth.

Psychoanalysis is by far most concerned with suffering that arises from our many internal divisions. Playfully, it is a form of deep brain stimulation. It focuses not only on our relationships with others but also on our relationships with ourselves and/or the others within us. It also attempts to distinguish historical writing from more or less arbitrary 'hystorical' falsification.

12 Better and Wiser: The Outcome

In a one-liner, psychotherapy can be defined as using our thinking to understand our feelings. Gaining a more holistic knowledge of our affairs ensures that the person concerned can better lead their life to the fullest.

The French writer Michel Houellebecq once said in an interview: *ultimately, life breaks our hearts*. Psychoanalyst Wilfred Bion replies laconically when given a fatal prognosis: *life is full of surprises, most of them unpleasant*. Or, more plastically expressed, I quote Kurt Cobain, the singer-songwriter of Nirvana: *nobody dies a virgin; life fucks us all*. Psychoanalysis does not make us immune to ordinary human misery, but it does contribute to increasing our resilience even in the face of the harshest facts of life. It is not entirely neutral because it is in the service of life, not only in its biological (of mere survival) but especially in its existential meaning.

The patients who now have their say shed light on what occurs in our darkest valleys. They have all experienced 'no pain, no gain' to a greater or lesser extent. When my publisher asked what struck me most, I replied that they feel better and wiser through psychotherapy – most even better and wiser than ever. What a – this time pleasant – surprise! I thank them for the trust, courage and candour with which they went through their process and bear witness.

Chapter 3

Patient Testimonies

1 A.B.

On their honeymoon in Italy, my parents watched the live coverage of the first men on the moon together. Two years later, I was born. As the first grandchild on my mother's side, I was warmly welcomed and thrived. My parents, active in education, started building their own house in my first years. As a craftsman, my father spent all his free time with knowledge and skill in constructing, finishing, and embellishing our house and garden. From him, I received my technical and practical insight, a sense of design, aesthetics and perseverance.

Unfortunately, the many hours of work and family life – my younger brother joined us after moving into the new house – did not prevent my father from regularly drinking too much and staying away from home. As the years went by, this took on increasingly more significant proportions. His abusive tirades under the influence often kept us awake for hours and, sometimes, we were startled in the middle of the night by his arrival home, the time of which was impossible to predict. The relationship between my father and mother was under increasing pressure. Due to his violent and threatening behaviour, my mother frequently called on the help of the doctor or the police, and sometimes she sent me and/or my brother to a neighbour because we were so afraid of being alone with him and in the hope that a third person could calm him down somewhat. We fled the house – even at night – and then slept at a relative's home. Then we had to quickly get our clothes and school bags ready with everything for the next day and try to leave the house so that he wouldn't notice.

This situation that dominated our family life lasted for years, with many small and a few significant crises. In the year the Berlin Wall fell, my father was in a detoxification clinic. My brother went to boarding school, and I found myself on the threshold of adulthood as the man of the house. The detoxification process took several years, during which my father was admitted a second time and then moved into accommodation in the grounds of the clinic. The family – his wife and children – seemed of secondary importance to him. He

DOI: 10.4324/9781003528067-3

also kept us in the dark about whether he wanted to return home and when. Sometimes, he came home briefly but only to be occupied with his leisure activities; there was no conversation. The parental responsibility of running the household and caring for the home and garden was not his forte. So, that responsibility fell on me, including emotional involvement towards my mother.

These were also the years I began exploring the world and going out with friends. My father finally retired when we were both still studying, but as far as we could tell, he was now finally able to give up drinking. He found a second wind in the launch and rural development of a guild for crafts, and very slowly, the trust between my parents was also restored. I had already started my descent into hell, and it would cost me twenty of my best years to reach that low point, where I felt and knew and dared to admit to myself that I could no longer function with alcohol and not without it either. Then there is only one way out, and that is death; it was just a matter of time if I kept drinking because I took enormous risks under the influence of alcohol and had already narrowly escaped several times.

My detoxification was a process of falling and getting up. During and in the aftermath of the banking crisis, I was job-seeking for about nine months. Although things went further downhill, it was also in this period that the foundations for my later recovery were laid, thanks to the conversations with the familiar psychologist I had seen at intervals since a car accident and the first conversations with a psychiatrist. After yet another relapse into alcohol and without a job, I finally started to loathe myself. Then something awoke in me, though I can't possibly say what – an inner strength. After nearly forty years in life, a difficult childhood, no relationships formed, and much grief, fear and pain inflicted on my mother, father and brother, I still wanted to 'do something' with my life. Then I had to start on it. I saw the new job as a new start and slowly got myself back on track. Looking back, I see that period as the turning point.

At the start of my psychotherapeutic process, I had already been sober for over seven years. In overcoming my alcohol dependence, I was convinced that I managed, and what I experienced as feelings of discomfort, stress, frustrations towards work and relational problems, I continued to explain and accept for myself as the usual difficulties and setbacks of life that everyone sometimes has to deal with, and that much – if not everything – could be solved and would become more liveable if 'the other' would realise their mistake and adapt their behaviour. At a certain point, the inner tension had built up so high that I also developed physical complaints. The GP (general practitioner) (who was very willing to listen) referred me initially to a psychologist. What I saw as the cause of my problems, a toxic cocktail of work and relationship problems, I was able to articulate in a structured way with her, which initially helped. This period lasted about six months. Because I started to feel worse after a while and became over-stressed, the GP first prescribed two weeks of rest for me, followed by another two weeks. There was a very intense conversation with the doctor in which I also mentioned my previous visits to my psychiatrist; these had taken place years earlier, in the period just before and after I stopped drinking. With some reluctance, I suggested possibly getting back in touch with this psychiatrist. The GP strongly encouraged this and was unwilling to let me rest at home without more. I got an appointment very quickly. His advice was direct and challenging but also unambiguous. He proposed an in-depth approach, starting with a full-time admission to the clinical psychotherapeutic unit he headed in a psychiatric hospital. The prospect of being absent from work for a more extended period (at the time, I thought for a maximum of six to eight weeks) frightened me, but when I left his consulting room, I already knew that I just had to do this; there was no alternative left. I was indeed 'done for', felt very tired, and had a whole problematic history with periodic visits to a psychologist behind me. Indeed, this had put things in the right direction, but more was needed.

The introduction to the ward went exceptionally smoothly. The professionalism, calm, insight, understanding and humanity immediately touched me. I didn't have to explain much and had little to be ashamed of. There was an instant feeling of trust. I had excellent contact with my personal counsellor and the trainee psychologist, whom I could also see individually weekly alongside our ward psychologist. From the outset, everything was in place to work confidently and in-depth. The day and weekly programmes were well filled, built up of the fixed blocks in which you participate as a treatment group member, with the 'forum' activities that I could partly fill in myself. I never felt that the days were too busy; it was just right, but it was progressing. With some distance, the treatment was well considered, well thought-out, and flexible so that the patient's needs for recovery were optimally met. It is mainly about speaking, expressing in a non-harmful way and a protected environment, emotional content that I had until then tried to master in a harmful and destructive way for myself – and those around me.

Self-expression is much broader than individual or group discussions. There is, for example, the therapy of pictorial expression, music therapy, movement therapy, etc. It is exceptional to establish something you did not yet know was in you through a simple assignment and your creativity, as well as the emergence of new insights through the subsequent discussion and the reactions of fellow patients to your work.

The various therapies and supporting forum activities aim to encourage you to speak, which has worked well for me. I have always seen my individual therapeutic contacts as helpful, open and honest. Speaking during group psychotherapy has taught me to dare to express my feelings and thoughts, take positions and defend them, even in the presence of 'third parties'. The course of these group psycho-sessions was always unpredictable and often very intense for the speaker and/or for one or more listeners in the group. By the end of the programme, I could have taken the floor more, but I learned an enormous amount from listening carefully to others and observing the reactions within the group. Although it was not foreseeable at the programme's start, I spent the entire first period in full-time admission. I came back to breathe, and that stability gave me a solid basis to dare to take steps during the therapy sessions and interview moments. I could spend the weekend and Wednesday afternoons freely and, during this period, I also arranged my change of residence and move. After a while, I started to experience the clinic as my new home. It felt like a safe and warm environment. This was discussed, and because I knew rationally that this situation could not last too long (and because my evolution was favourable), I started my second period in daycare after trial leave.

The transition went smoothly; the treatment did not change, and the activities and interview moments continued. This period was at least as necessary and fruitful as the first; I saw fellow patients evolve and receive positive comments from others, sometimes also about myself. I couldn't quite put my finger on it, but I felt that something was changing within me. I have fond and beautiful memories of my stay and look back on it with nostalgia.

A combination of day clinic and gradual return to work characterised my third period. At the same time, I started weekly visits to a psychologist-psychotherapist in private practice. The extra travel was a bit more complex, and it also weighed on me that I could no longer fully follow the weekly programme; I felt I was missing something and no longer fully part of what had become dear to me in the meantime: the therapies, the people and the environment. Here, too, I was confronted with myself again. The gradual work went quite well, and I knew I was progressing towards a full return.

I had undertaken a very adventurous and active group trip between periods two and three. I was able to start something new and, above all, make good contacts and feel a connection with others. With those recharged batteries and backed by the team, I completed the treatment and resumed my work full-time. I continued to see the psychologist weekly and the psychiatrist monthly. After about six months, I put the consultations with the psychologist on hold, but I have not resumed them since. I continued to see the doctor monthly for follow-up, and this continued until the start of the coronavirus epidemic. I did not take up the option of online consultations.

For a long time, I had the feeling and conviction that my stay in the clinic and the treatment there had brought about a stable and lasting change, and this was certainly the case the first time after my discharge. Last year, however, there have been several isolated cases of relapse into alcohol use, after which a period of almost daily use with sometimes larger quantities. I also started to feel more and more tired, as well as experiencing more muscle aches. I contacted the GP and started a relaxation therapy/physiotherapy treatment. The positive energy, warm personality and very intense initial exploratory conversation motivated me naturally to stop the alcohol; at the time of writing this, I am still doing well with that.

The sessions with the therapist are just as valuable to me as those I had with a psychologist or psychotherapist, but it was a very sobering surprise to find that there is still a lot to 'process'. I am again dealing with fatigue, muscle tension and sometimes negative thoughts, and the previous alcohol consumption has functioned as a blanket to numb my pains and calm my mind. Now it's all back: I'm overstimulated, quickly tired, and can no longer relax. In my feeling, it is so that my body and mind still hold a lot of grief, pain and loss and that I have to tackle this again. It should be mentioned that my father died less than two years ago; it now feels as if he has never left and is even more insistently present.

I also want to shed some light on my experiences with women – other than my mother. As a child, I was very good friends with N., a girl from the street who was one year younger. We grew up together. As a teenager, she started friendships with other boys she knew from school. She confided in me about her 'relationships' with them – her crushes and heartbreaks. It hurt me because I was secretly in love with her and couldn't find a way to express it, but I still felt special because she continued to see me as her primary support alongside her girlfriends. As we grew older, the contact diminished. At college, I met K. We were both a bit withdrawn and found each other in friendship. She could drink heavily and was no less of a man than any other. She was a good student, though, and we motivated each other to catch up on missed lessons after one of us had skipped a class. But she fell in love with the barman …

Also, during these student years, I lapsed into a kind of coma after consuming large amounts of alcohol at a dorm party and woke up in the emergency department. To my great surprise, it turned out that I had hooked up with I. that evening. She was and remained convinced that we were a couple, but I – and to this day – could remember nothing of that evening, and it cost me much effort to make her understand that our 'relationship' was a big mistake.

Years later, I started visiting prostitutes. I only met them in hotels. One girl (A.) especially struck me from the first meeting, and we made a second appointment. It remained just talking that hour, but I found that anything but unpleasant; there was mutual understanding and trust. We continued to see each other, sometimes several times a week, and we chatted endlessly. I was hopelessly in love, but she was in a relationship. Still, we continued to meet. This lasted about ten months. In the summer, she went on holiday with her boyfriend, and afterwards, there was no more contact, although we exchanged a few text messages. During this period, I sometimes made another appointment with a young lady, which led to intimacy. In the following years, I continued to visit prostitutes regularly.

At work, I met E., a female colleague. When I first saw her, something strange went through me. She was new and eager to learn; I shared my professional knowledge. From one thing came another, and we quickly became a couple. It was my first real relationship. But E. was dealing with many fears herself; I was happy to be a listening ear. In the relationship, I often took on a caring role; later, a work-related problem was added. The ties came under increasing pressure, and we both sought professional help, but that could not save the relationship. We are still colleagues, and there is mutual respect and warm contact, but we no longer see each other outside of work.

A few weeks after the start of my clinical psychotherapeutic admission, I met someone for the first time again who could touch me (V.). She came from a distant country, was temporarily here, and had ended up in this 'work' and missed her six-year-old daughter, who had remained with her parents. When making a new appointment, I sometimes stood before a closed door but didn't give up. In the year-end period, she would return to her home country, and because her daughter's birthday was also in that period, I bought some toys (including a colouring book and a doctor's set because she would like to become one later). Later, she sent me a photo of her daughter in that doctor's coat. I enjoyed being with her; we both enjoyed a moment of relaxation, and how we filled the intimate moments was entirely suitable for me. However, I didn't want to keep seeing her in a conditional – paid – way because I had learned from earlier experiences, and my financial situation also forced me a bit in that direction. Still, I didn't come to a clear message to her. We continued to stay in touch by phone, even a few years after our last meeting. At one point, she asked for financial help, and I pushed for a – regular – meeting, but she kept her distance. She said she was seriously ill. Afterwards, the contact faded out.

During my last treatment, I became fascinated by a fellow patient, S., who was not part of my group. She was in a clear state of emotional weakness for me, and she avoided any attempt at contact. Trust and respect grew after a few months and through the evening sports opportunities in the clinic. As I got to know her better, I fell in love, although I saw no possibility of doing anything with it. She was also in a relationship. Still, after a while, she felt for herself what I felt for her, and we had a long and intense conversation. By how she treated me and the message she brought that a relationship was impossible, my respect and affection for her grew, as well as the conviction that I was still capable of an honest and genuine deep human relationship. But she was not free, and that hit me so hard that I wanted to stop everything, even my life. That evening, I drank, and she helped me through it via the phone and lots of messages. I will always be grateful to her for that. After our stay in the centre, we remained in touch, and now, a few years later, we still have a good connection.

This year, I have also fallen passionately in love with someone who is not free. Never before has someone been able to touch me so quickly and so profoundly. Sometimes, I realise that a pattern is emerging in my love life. I am condemned to being a confidant and caring for a woman in trouble. However, I still don't see it clearly and want to analyse it further.

2 A.G.

My life's a tangled mess, and I've unravelled quite a few threads, but I haven't been able to cut them. It's probably *because* I am a tangled mess. My half-sister is on my father's side, and I'm the elder of two daughters. I think my parents' relationship was always turbulent. My father drank and was aggressive, and my mother often had to flee with us, sleeping at various addresses. I still remember the shouting and screaming and one scene where my father threw a hammer at my mother's head. I often lay quietly in my bed, my heart pounding, waiting for him to burst into my bedroom. Once I had to go to hospital for a head wound. I think my father hit me. Or did I fall against the fridge? We often had to go looking for my dad in pubs with Mum. Sometimes, I was tasked with getting him home, but even then, he'd continue drinking pints with his friends while I sat waiting with an empty glass. I fear my glass is still empty. My only happy childhood memories are from my maternal grandparents; I could be a child and play there.

Around the age of ten, my parents separated. We stayed with my mother, and after a period of material comfort, several years of financial hardship, bailiffs and misery followed. My father had many girlfriends. Some were kind to us, others not at all. He hospitalised a couple of them. There was no fixed visitation schedule. Essentially, my father barely looked at us. Things were often difficult with Mum. As a single mother, she had a hard time and could be very quick-tempered, even physically harsh. Our house was a tip. It was just dirty and disgusting. I was ashamed and didn't dare invite friends over. At school, I often felt inferior, bullied or excluded. This got worse in secondary school when I was hurt and humiliated because of my clothes and appearance. During break time, I often retreated to the toilets. I escaped into books or a fantasy world where I paired up with Harry Potter or the lead singer of a boy band. Around that age, however, I already had suicidal thoughts and started cutting my arms. I quickly learned not to talk to Mum and tried to fend for myself. Around sixteen, I found a local pub where I felt at home. I adopted a punk image and started giving the finger and talking back, which made the bullies at school leave me alone. I did all sorts of things I shouldn't have: shoplifting, drinking, sleeping with one boy after another. I used sex and my body to get some love and attention, but I was often dumped or felt dumped. Because of my behaviour, I lost the few friends I had. My first serious boyfriend lived on the other side of the country. He was into drugs, a bad boy who cheated on me with his ex from the start, but I had to have him! We had a turbulent on-off relationship, where he heavily flirted with other girls. I was always afraid he would abandon me, but I was also furious and jealous, so I constantly checked up on him. In the end, he dumped me like a piece of trash.

I pursued higher education in youth care and learned much from the lessons. I had alternative looks by then and felt increasingly valued and recognised. On the other hand, I kept ending up in relationships that weren't good for me. Looking back, I was mainly looking for security, but always with the same type: bastards. Around twenty, I was emotionally exhausted and took an overdose of my mother's antidepressants. It was mainly a cry for help and the first step on a long road to recovery. I was admitted to a psychiatric ward. I thought I'd find peace and safety there, but it was anything but. I sabotaged the therapies, smoked weed in the park, stayed in bed and started self-harming more and more seriously than ever before. This led to me being transferred to a secure ward. The boundaries I was given there (I sometimes asked to be put in seclusion) did me good and gradually calmed me down. I desperately needed a clear and safe framework. I stayed there for several months. I don't remember much from the therapies or conversations there, except for one specific session with the psychologist. I had to represent our family with dolls, and I remember throwing my father out of the window and putting myself on an equal footing with my mother. I didn't realise the significance at the time, but now I realise that (probably out of revenge) I've thrown away many men, and, as the eldest daughter, I more than adequately took on the mother role. Around that time, my older half-sister reappeared after many years. She visited me in the hospital with a book I cherish: *The Solitude of Prime Numbers*. I find it a beautiful (and highly relatable!) title. Towards the end of that admission, I met H., a friend's ex – and my friend was very angry that I had started a relationship with him. I was really into H. He seemed like my saviour. He came from a good, stable home, and I thought I'd found my soulmate. With him, I started drinking occasionally (too much) for fun. H. moved in with us, but when my mother got a new partner, she clarified that we had to leave. We moved out, I started working, and the problems began. He was an absolute control freak. Everything had to be orderly and tidy, and when it wasn't to his liking, he could become very volatile and even physically abusive. I also didn't feel good in my skin, had gained several kilos and felt increasingly insecure. I escaped into a relationship with a colleague but felt very guilty about it at the same time. I started having eating problems, became fixated on my food and the scales, and sought a sense of security and control over them. All in all, I experienced a few years of reasonable stability. I contacted my father, wanting to discuss various things with him. I sought understanding and recognition and hoped he would apologise and take responsibility. He didn't. He had zero empathy or feeling, and I wondered if I also had such a 'bad' character. The relationship with H. became more difficult again. He became increasingly verbally aggressive, and I suggested relationship therapy. He was furious about that. We decided to have a child, hoping it would improve our relationship. During my pregnancy, I felt great, but H. was difficult. Arguments about all sorts of things I wasn't doing right in the household became commonplace, and I repeatedly fled in tears to my mother. The birth of our daughter was a cold shower. I wasn't on cloud nine, which I thought I'd be on. In no time at all, I was completely physically and emotionally exhausted. H. barely took on the father role and, instead of supporting me, H. abandoned me. Our relationship also went downhill sexually. I had absolutely no libido. Meanwhile, my mother had started a relationship, and it was the same old story. Her boyfriend drank, cheated on her and was aggressive. I couldn't handle all that misery. I threatened to cut off all contact with her if she stayed with that bastard. During that period, I had a conversation with my younger sister where I detailed what I had to endure from H.: not only verbal but sometimes also physical violence, humiliation and death threats. The fact that my sister used the words 'domestic violence' has stayed with me, but I still can't call it that. I thought I was flawed and deserved to be treated so badly. Still, something gradually broke, and my intention to separate from H. became increasingly firm. We've been separated for almost ten years now, and I can say that we are 'happily separated'. There will be no more conflicts, and we can communicate well, make agreements, and cooperate with our daughter.

Shortly after the break-up with H., I met B. He is eighteen years older than me and the father of two children. He was separating when I met him. He was the first man who paid me so much sexual care and attention, and we initially had an excellent and passionate relationship. It all happened very quickly. We moved in together quickly, and I soon found myself in a challenging and complex blended family with his children and my daughter, where we had little (literal and figurative) space. There was also a return of jealousy and control, with B.'s staying out late and occasional alcohol consumption triggering me. B. also carried a past with many relationship and emotional problems. There were problems at work, and both my mother and my younger sister were struggling psychologically, requiring me to step in often and help. I felt cornered and started acting difficult towards B. He couldn't do anything right; I started drinking a lot and became like H. in my relationship: arguments, accusations, humiliation, outbursts of anger. I was full of negative feelings that I was taking out on him. I started to feel like the abuser. I started acting as severely as my father or H. B. distanced himself, trying to make it clear to me that I had serious psychiatric problems. I was beyond reason. Eventually, B. fled into the arms of a neighbour. I almost chased him away but only really went mad when I realised he was cheating on me. I was distraught and made a mess of everything. When B. ended the relationship, I collapsed. I had lost everything, and it was all my fault. Instead of remaining constructive, I acted like a bitch in every way. I moved in with my mother for a while. I was a wreck, drank myself silly, and did almost nothing outside of work. Sometimes, I tried to seduce B. and win him back; other times, I acted horribly. I went on Tinder and started dating and hooking up with several men. I was utterly emotionally distraught and just acted out. I felt scared, lost and guilty, and eventually made a serious suicide attempt. I considered myself an absolute monster who deserved the death penalty. I was admitted to a psychiatric ward again, but it didn't help much. After many more months of on-and-off rapprochement and distance from B., I started psychotherapy with my current psychiatrist. I've been seeing him weekly for about a year-and-a-half. From the start, he went into my life history in great detail. We have a LAT ('living apart together') relationship, but B. and I have much more peace. Sexually, I keep my distance, but the feeling of safety and trust is being restored. We both acknowledge our roles in the turbulence of our relationship. Shortly after starting psychotherapy, I gained a clearer understanding of my problems. The tangled mess I mentioned initially consists of several recurring, identifiable threads. I try to unravel them further each week. Firstly, I have a significant attachment problem. I quickly feel unsafe and abandoned, and I try to escape those feelings by drowning them in a few glasses of alcohol. This problem is now largely under control. Self-harm is a thing of the past. I have a problem with my self-image and self-worth. I wasn't worth anything to my father. I exhaust myself for men, especially sexually, but I always get a hang-over from those efforts, and then sadness, anger and defiance surface. Can I trust and rely on my partner? Especially with B., there's a revenge factor at work. I want to make him pay for all the pain inflicted on me by my father and other men. Sometimes, I play with his … and sometimes, I enjoy belit-tling, scaring or humiliating him. It seems as if I want to reverse the roles and make him feel the pain I've experienced as a woman. I try to do well for my daughter and the troubled young people at work. Caring for others is cer-tainly something I've wanted to do since childhood, for my mother and both my sisters. I was largely left to my own devices but also had much freedom. I could get my way a lot and find it difficult when confronted with authority. However, I benefit from some boundaries and guidance if I feel sufficiently respected and heard. This is something I was almost completely lacking in my youth. As far as I can judge, my daughter is doing well. I work full-time and get a lot of freedom and responsibility in a dual role as an experience-worker and coordinator for young people in need. How my relationship will continue is still unclear. Now that I'm in therapy, I'm also trying to convince B. to go into psychotherapy. I'm working on my contribution to our relationship pro-blems. The question is whether he can or is willing to reflect on himself.

3 A.N.

I am now a woman in my late forties and have my act together reasonably well. I was born on the other side of the world to a Belgian mother and a local father. My mother was his seventh (!) wife, and I am (until now anyway) '*known*' as his seventh child – perhaps his eighth. When I was four, my mother returned to the Netherlands with me and my younger sister. I grew up there in a very violent environment: abuse, sexual abuse, emotional, material (shabby clothes, too little or spoilt food) and pedagogical (one didn't let me do any-thing, and the other didn't look after me) neglect. Rules were set by my step-father so strictly and at the same time arbitrarily that I could not comply with them. He watched me constantly so that I felt both controlled and terrorised by him. I was 'the ugly duckling in the bite' nobody could do anything with, so he would raise that on his own. Luckily, grandma and grandpa were there. On top of that, my 'parents' were both alcohol-addicted with an evil temper.

From the age of seventeen to nineteen, I was admitted to a psychoanalytic community for adolescents. Psychoanalysis in therapeutic practice was in its infancy at that time, especially for children and adolescents. During that period, I was cutting and scratching my skin open. Eventually, I graduated from high school. I spent two years there, found some safety and footing, and obtained a bachelor's degree in social work. I worked non-stop for the next five years and lived with my first partner. This did not work out, so I met my current ex-partner. We have three adolescent children together, have been divorced for six years, and get along wonderfully as parents.

After admission, I was doing moderately to reasonably well. I met my Belgian partner while travelling in Nepal, burned my lot in the Netherlands and went to live in Belgium. I wanted a nice family life: partner, children, house and a good job. I had a lovely daughter and a big son, and, over ten years ago, after a difficult pregnancy and a planned Caesarean section, our youngest son was born. I remember thinking then: it's over. This was my goal, and now what? I then breastfed for another nine months, with no sleep and constant reliving of the numerous traumas of my childhood. My children no longer had a mum. Depression is a strange beast. They were still tiny when I entered admission. What I expected from it was to be out, healed and well as soon as possible to resume my mother, partner and employee duties and be admitted for as short a time as possible. The 'surgery' could not go fast enough for me.

The first admission lasted seventeen months in full hospitalisation and later day therapy. After this, I was in progressive employment for eighteen months, re-experiencing trauma again, but this time of a different and heavier calibre. Thereafter, I had several short, twenty-four-hour- or day-therapy admissions until I was diagnosed with Type II bipolar disorder following a euphoric and agitated hyperactive phase. After a full-blown manic psychosis a year later, I was 'upgraded' to bipolar disorder Type I. In retrospect, these states had a lot to do with a kind of flight forward after my partner abandoned me because of lingering problems and treatment. Since then, I have been fighting, rebounding and trying to live an everyday, calm life with healthy stress with the help of post-cure inpatient treatment and from my psychiatrist, but it is a difficult road.

I always preferred to ignore do-therapies. I am not creatively inclined, nor does it 'tell' me anything. Making collages, drawing and beating a drum was an absolute waste of my time. Nevertheless, I have a good (verbal) relationship with those therapists. 'Milieu therapy' does nothing for me! All those 'disturbed' people, and they are by far my best contacts now! As mentioned, expressive therapies did not suit me. I was downright moody during expressive therapy and questioned music therapy out loud, although I was thrilled when I or someone else played a song. I dared to sit behind the piano with the therapist during individual music therapy. Still, I imposed on myself the standard that it had to be 'beautiful', which never went out in both music and expressive therapy. I am more of a speaker, so group psychotherapy and process guidance suited me better. I have experienced several therapy groups in over a decade of clinical psychotherapy. And my conclusion is that everyone has to fight for their place. To speak up, engage in recognition and make connections. And sometimes, it doesn't click at all. And then you are a 'bird for the cat'. Then you get spat out by the group, and you must continue working individually. I hope the group eventually accepts you back.

As I mentioned earlier, I didn't get much out of non-verbal therapies. I could never play during my childhood; if you can do this, you will be more prepared. I am a very rational person. Modelling and colouring did not suit me at all. Eventually, I'd manage to clay my most considerable trauma in the creative studio. Why? Because there were no demands, and I was allowed to do what I wanted. Process guidance was also crucial for me. In the first part of my treatment, twice a week, and later, once a week. It is essential to map/ bring your process, hear about others and understand where they are in their process. After all these years, I realised that the therapeutic process for patients goes down bumpy roads. Sometimes, you suddenly have new insights and make steps forward, only to stand still for a while. The same happens with your fellow patients. This is almost a give-and-take, coming-and-going.

After more than a decade, I am still in psychotherapy with my psychiatrist (I am still not allowed to call him by first name) and cannot say when it will end. Over the years, there have been several shifts: from the frightened, anxious child to someone who (sometimes with much effort) can take on everyday life again. In the form of now single parenthood, performing my job as a social assistant and my contribution to society, it was with a lot of trial and error and (often with help) getting up. Unfortunately, many partners, family members and friends drop out of this process because it takes too long. My trauma, however, also took far too long. I am lucky that the psychiatrist came my way; otherwise, I wouldn't be alive anymore. I hope he continues to practise and doesn't become deaf and/or demented (his words) for a long time to come.

I have long since lost expectations for the future. Processing a psycho-traumatic past is hard work for years. You take it day by day. After over a decade of admission, I did not work for long periods. As a result, I lost all credit with my employer and was targeted more and more (like by my step-father at the time). Eventually, my employer and I could no longer get along. But because I always stayed at work between admissions, I managed to retain my skills and expertise and, despite my age, I proved to be a sought-after person in the job market. It also overwhelmed me that I quickly found a new job that satisfied me more than the previous one. After all, it allows me to renew my social commitment.

4 B.S.

It started with depressive symptoms, a feeling of not being well in my skin. Looking back, I felt like I didn't belong, even as a child. I gave off too few signals that I was there alongside my brother. I have trouble forming more profound relationships and expressing my anger. The latter started as a toddler when I pushed my brother hard against a cupboard, after which I was sidelined while my mother took my brother to the doctor. At that point, I probably repressed all my aggression, which only surfaced later in intense outbursts when my 'cup' was full. In lower secondary school, this led to me being bullied. Because of this, I had a restricted adolescence because I didn't want to detach myself from my only anchor: home. During the four-month training of my national service, I was bullied again.

When I was first made redundant after a year of work, I went to the GP with depressive symptoms. With medication and finding a new job, I got better. After a few years, things deteriorated again. Then, in addition to drugs, my GP gave me an appointment with a behavioural psychologist. Because this didn't help, he referred me to another psychologist. She immediately referred me to a psychotherapist. I was lucky that my GP and that psychologist referred me quickly and effectively. My GP also had a conversation with me at every consultation. When I lost my second job after eight years, things got worse again, and the sessions with the psychotherapist were no longer sufficient. Although I had found new work in the meantime, the supportive medication didn't help either, and then my GP referred me to a psychotherapeutic ward in a psychiatric hospital.

Due to a two-year admission, I ultimately lost this job as well. Fortunately, I was still secretary of an amateur theatre group. After a few years, there was disagreement within the board, and I resigned. Through volunteering, I ended up in a completely different job, far less suited to my competencies and university degree. In this new organisation, I was initially able to grow somewhat, but soon, my opportunities and competencies were curtailed. Recently, I was made redundant there, too.

My first psychologist/psychotherapist gave me a good explanation of what psychotherapy is and how it works. Because of this, you don't have high expectations, and it works better, especially in the beginning. In group therapy, the stories of others sometimes bring about associations that you don't get in individual treatment. Furthermore, you also develop relationships with the other people in the group.

In total, I have been in psychotherapy for over twenty years. This is because it's a fundamental problem deeply ingrained. When you're not admitted, you also miss 'here-and-now' sessions and therapies, making it harder to change your situation. You receive little positive feedback. You mostly get only negative feedback from your environment because they don't want you to change. And you are insecure about tackling things differently. You lose contact with the people around you. After my admission, my brother broke off all contact with me. Contact has since been restored.

In psychotherapy, you discover what lies behind your problem and where it comes from. But that doesn't solve it. And that's precisely the most challenging part. For that, there should be a kind of follow-up and support for 'here-

and-now' issues in addition to psychotherapy, especially if you have few people around you. When you're admitted, it's said that you can 'practise' with fellow patients. However, the problem is that they are also struggling with themselves, so they don't react like people outside the clinic. On the other hand, you can safely learn things. It didn't work out for me to try a more intimate relationship because it wasn't mutual.

During my admission, I started living independently, which allowed me to detach myself from my parents better. I also became more assertive but not yet (positively) aggressive enough. Because of that, I still fall by the wayside too much. I now hope to find a good job that will make me more self-confident. Relationships will then also work out better.

5 B.W.

As a child and adolescent, I already received many signals that I was insecure and anxious. For example, I could be afraid of a man with a beard for no reason, or I would have to vomit before a presentation or exam. I was often restless and reacted more emotionally than my environment in certain situations. Panic was a normal reaction for me to most 'problems'. I didn't understand those signals then or even know what stress was. I just lived from one moment of anxiety to the next; fortunately, I could still enjoy many carefree years in between.

It wasn't until I started working after my higher education that anxiety and stress became a daily occurrence. After a relationship breakdown, I completely fell apart. I neglected my work, and the slightest effort cost me enormous energy. Even a simple ballpoint pen was too heavy to lift. It's hard to believe, but that's how listless I felt. I saw my future gloomily. Did I have to keep doing this work until retirement? Would I ever experience love again? Nothing made sense anymore; I cancelled all my appointments and ongoing projects. I thought this reduction in workload would ease my suffering, but instead, I felt guilty and cowardly, completely incompetent. I was twenty-three then and realised it couldn't go on like this. In the first phase, I still looked for a physical cause. I had a stomach examination and took Motilium for nausea and aspirin for headaches, but my physical symptoms remained.

The relationship breakdown continued to linger. I often worried during the day, cried frequently, slept poorly, had no appetite and ended up in a psychotic episode for the first time. I thought everyone was speaking badly about me, laughing at me or trying to bring me down. Full of suspicion and distrust, I lost all sense of reality. Even though I usually paid attention to my clothing and personal hygiene, I 'forgot' to wash, shave or put on fresh clothes. I didn't eat or sleep anymore, couldn't focus on a book or film, and didn't dare go shopping anymore. I wandered the streets and toyed with the idea of committing suicide so that everything would finally be over.

Shortly afterwards, my first admission to a psychiatric hospital followed. I don't remember how I ended up there, but it was just in time because, despite the medication, my condition was getting worse. I didn't trust anyone and even thought that the hospital staff wanted to lure me into a trap. I checked every room for hidden cameras, and my mind spun like never before. At one point, I was convinced that, like Jesus Christ, I had stigmata on my feet and palms, but apparently, I was the only one who saw these red marks. A severe identity crisis had set in. I doubted everything and everyone, but most of all myself. After my discharge from the hospital, I went to a psychiatrist weekly, but he only wanted to know if I was eating and sleeping well while the inner conflicts, unrest, and self-doubt were draining my body and life.

On the advice of a family member, I ended up with another psychiatrist who immediately asked completely different questions. I didn't understand why it had to be about my parents and childhood. What did this have to do with my current psychosomatic complaints? The psychotherapist also said very little while I almost begged for a diagnosis. What's wrong with me? Am I manic-depressive? Do I have borderline personality disorder? Am I schizo-phrenic? The doctor didn't answer such questions. He listened and remained silent; occasionally, he nodded. I remember always leaving the first sessions angry because I felt the man had quickly earned money. Only after some time did I realise that my problems originated in the past. Yet, I didn't immediately feel helped; on the contrary, the psychotherapy was very confronting, and my mind was fully occupied between sessions with analysing and processing the things I had just discovered about myself or my past. There was no more room in my head for other things, so I forgot essential appointments, dates or names. I lost my concentration both privately and at work. I could spend hours worrying and losing myself in thoughts that didn't match reality. I dreamt of leaving everything behind (house, car, work, family, friends, …) and fleeing abroad to lead a vagrant existence. A new psychosis was developing; admission was inevitable.

While my first admission was relatively short (a few weeks), and I was helped back on my feet with medication, my second admission was long-term (more than a year), and I received more psychotherapy and less medication. By now, I was used to individual therapy, but it was a high hurdle to expose myself in group sessions as well. I also doubted whether I was in the right place. Those other patients seemed to have experienced much worse things than I had … Because I didn't have to work anymore, much stress fell off me, and I could fully concentrate on my therapy. I did suffer from shame; 'psy-chiatric patient' was not a label that my ego could bear, and I felt guilty towards my employer and colleagues whom I had 'let down'. After a while, I was able to attend day therapy, and then outpatient treatment was increased to two sessions per week. I felt that I had gained quality of life and had lived rather superficially before my psychotherapy. I understood myself and others better and thought I was 'fully healed'.

Yet, the stress quickly returned as soon as I resumed my work. Soon, I was back in a cycle of daily vomiting. Although I could probably hide it well, I continuously suffered from a fear of failure and was afraid that I would lose my job and wouldn't be able to pay off my house. However, the most tremendous losses manifested themselves relationally. My relationships started passionately but ended after a few weeks or months. I had romantic ideals in my head and quickly gave up on them when the blue sky began to show clouds. After every relationship breakdown, I was left disappointed, hurt and confused. This probably applied equally to my exes. I didn't know what I wanted. As a single person, I wanted a relationship as quickly as possible, and as soon as I was in a relationship, I longed for a single life again. I was never satisfied with my results in work and hobbies, while others praised my achievements. It took fifteen years of therapy before I could let go of a certain perfectionism, but what a relief that not everything has to be perfect.

I no longer have to prove myself; I no longer have to be the best; I am good enough. It was a matter of getting used to this 'new me' for me and my environment. I knew how far down I had come and considered every day of work accomplished a victory, while my employer wanted to raise the bar. I like to compare it to someone who was in a wheelchair and is grateful that they can walk again, but no one should expect them to start running again immediately. My emotions and thoughts, partly due to getting older, have become milder and gentler for myself and others. Heaven and hell, the stormy rivers of yesteryear, have given way to an earthly, meandering stream.

Despite these psychological changes, I was still not spared from depression, burnout, and psychoses in the following decades. There were several periods of sick leave and hospital admissions, each with a few better years in between. Just before each admission, despite the many insights I gained, I had not a shred of awareness of illness. It's my family who brings me to the hospital because I'm showing the same symptoms again, no longer in reality. The admissions are short but no less intense for that. I still lose myself in far-reaching thoughts where I suspect conspiracies or think I'm someone else.

Jesus Christ has, therefore, risen several times, and I also imagined myself in the skin or the vicinity of several other religious or historical figures. I don't always know what happened or what I was daydreaming about. My imagination then runs away with me, and gaps appear in my short-term memory. I imagine that I am the cause of natural disasters or deaths. I can communicate with well-known world leaders without a phone. Not infrequently, I also hear voices or see objects come alive. (By the way, I have never used illegal drugs.)

During each admission, I think it will never get better for me, that I will never be able to resume my work, and that my partner will leave me because I live in another world. Fortunately, I have now been together with a lovely woman for more than ten years who has not let me down when I was struggling, even though it was not always easy for her to deal with my mental state. Currently, I take preventive medication: an antidepressant in the morning and an antipsychotic in the evening, and I regularly see a psychiatrist. My condition is stable, but I cannot predict how it will develop in the future despite all the therapy and medication. I hope I don't get sick again; that's all I can say. And yes, I sleep and eat well. That turns out to be more critical than I thought as a twenty-something.

Even though after twenty-five years of treatment, I can still have difficult moments, days or even weeks, I want to advise everyone struggling with mental health problems to work on it actively. Staying at home on sick leave won't get you anywhere. Use these temporary circumstances to work on yourself. In one way or another, those crisis periods and accompanying admissions have also been a blessing, the path to a better life, to a better me. Psychotherapy is not a wasted investment. Don't forget that you must spend your whole life, day and night, with yourself, so you might as well ensure you are in pleasant company. That last sentence might sound a bit schizophrenic, but we don't think so.

6 C.B.

'It's all about my birthday' was the first performance I created after graduating from dance school. Consciously or unconsciously, it expressed a deep-seated sense of loss I'd felt throughout my life: not being seen by my parents. My birthday was always an afterthought during a busy time of year for them. Little effort was made to celebrate it compared to my older brother and younger sister. I always felt caught in the middle, barely seen or heard. This probably drove me to the stage, developing my love for dance and performance. My body and mind could express what I thought and felt, things I couldn't articulate at home. The dance was my talent; others recognised and saw me through it.

I grew up in an unsafe family. My father was an alcoholic and, therefore, an absent caregiver. My mother tried her best to hold the family together but struggled mentally. My brother demanded enormous attention due to his unruly and aggressive behaviour. My sister and I endured his violence with little to no intervention from our parents. My sister and I tried to be as good as possible not to burden our parents further. In this way, we took on a caring role for them. Around the turn of the millennium, a computer and the internet entered the house. My father quickly found his way to porn websites, even when we children were at home. Seemingly wholly absorbed, he didn't seem to realise we witnessed him masturbating. My first experience with sexuality was utterly distorted. During my adolescence, my father also engaged in boundary-crossing behaviour, asking me, with mild coercion and payment, to massage him. At those times, I wasn't a child, a daughter, but a 'thing' that served him. The only way to keep those suppressed feelings and traumas under control was through controlling my food intake. Thin, thinnest, was my motto. It was a refusal to become a woman and, therefore, be available to men (my father, primarily). The world of dance reinforced this image: the thinner, the better, the more perfect, the more successful. These eating problems were a constant in my life since puberty, swinging from one extreme to the other and back again. I understood their origin and meaning only after intensive therapy, and the tension surrounding food has largely subsided.

As a child, I was well liked at school. My report cards repeatedly stated, 'C. is a ray of sunshine in the classroom'. I enjoyed studying and always did my best. However, I remember trying to keep my home problems secret at school from a very young age. I realised this was necessary to remain popular with my friends from seemingly perfect families. I had to project a good image of myself to fit in. A child doesn't betray their parents, I instinctively knew. Until I was twelve, I was burdened by the rigours of primary school, even one attended by nuns. Every Monday, the repeated question of who had been to church the previous day, the strict regime in the classrooms, corridors and refectory, the literal and figurative marching in step, and on top of that, children being forced to eat their vomit. Sexuality was a considerable taboo and not even discussed during the sex education classes. Sexuality was suppressed: good girls shouldn't show any interest in boys. Fortunately, the secondary school opened up a whole new world for me. I shared a school and classes with boys and discovered a more unrestrained way of thinking, with more room to develop myself. However, as the years went by, I felt increasingly depressed, reaching a peak around the age of sixteen. The problems at home became even more intense, and I couldn't or dared not talk to anyone about it. I kept all my thoughts and emotions bottled up inside. There was no possibility of venting at home. My signals were misinterpreted or ignored. I was alone. At school, I had no friends anymore; my classmates saw me as a strange person and became a target for bullying. My teachers also let me down. This starkly contrasted to the dance school, where I went several times a week. There, I was cherished for my talent. Two completely different worlds that seemed incompatible and led to confusion: Who was I? Only at university did the world truly open up for me; I finally felt at home, a world full of dance and like-minded people. I was no longer an outsider but fitted into a group of young people with the same passion, dreams and ambitions.

My parents separated during my second year at university. My father turned out to be gay, and my parents decided to divorce. My brother had known for years that my father was having an affair and had kept it to himself until the bomb exploded. And so a new taboo was born: we didn't talk about my father anymore because of how shameful it was to admit that our father was attracted to men despite having a broad and open outlook. My shame about the situation was so great that I could barely share it with anyone; it grew and consumed me. I felt like a shameful person, worthless, dirty, a zero. A lecturer once spoke to me to check on my well-being. That moment in the corridor at dance school marked the beginning of a long ordeal. I clung to him because he was the only one I could talk to about my feelings. But he abused his position of power, and I became his pawn, even in the direction of sexually boundary-crossing behaviour. Due to previous situations at home and not knowing what boundary-crossing behaviour was, I endured everything, assuming that this was just how it was and even my fault. Again, I felt deeply guilty, even dirtier and worthless. I couldn't turn to other students or lecturers; everything happened secretly. I felt obliged to remain silent, believing it was all my fault and that I had provoked everything. For the first time, I self-harmed by cutting my wrist. I often sought refuge in the woods, where a train rushed past at the edge. I imagined what it would be like to die there.

After graduating, I met a fellow student by chance. We spent our first year of university together and now live in the same city back in Belgium. We still connected well, fell in love, and married three years later. It felt like a good marriage where we were lovers and good friends. However, I barely realised or didn't realise at all, that I was being exploited in several ways. I took on a sizeable caring role and kept everything afloat. Sexually, he was demanding and, in the last years of our relationship, coercive. Again, there was my guilt: I was the one who never felt like having sex and, therefore, had a big problem. I had to change, and I had to meet his desires. It never occurred to me that I had the right to say 'no' and protect myself. Ten years ago, my depressive feelings intensified again after a few years of relative calm. I worked myself to death to avoid having to stop. I chased success and applause to feel some self-worth. At the same time, I often plummeted into despair when setbacks came my way. I only sought highs and sometimes allowed myself to be tempted by drugs. I was losing myself increasingly, unsure of who I was, where I came from, and how to react to my environment.

The entire therapeutic process began with visiting a sexologist with my husband, hoping to grow closer again and address 'my' sexual problem. Sometime later, I also consulted a psychologist because I felt I needed more support. I went weekly in some periods, sometimes every two weeks, some-times not at all for a while. I could talk about my daily worries, but it never led to a deep therapeutic process. Even during therapy, I tried to project a good image of myself. The shame of the events in my life was far too great. Besides, I genuinely believed life was hard, dark and depressing, and I had to make the best of it. Meanwhile, I continued to work hard, sometimes being away from home for weeks due to my work, undermining my health. A few years later, the ground suddenly disappeared from beneath my feet. Back home after a fierce confrontation with my husband, I fell to the ground and was unable to move. My body and mind shut down. After some time, I pulled myself up with a last bit of strength. I gathered all my courage to go out into the street and ring the doorbell of a nearby psychiatric institution. On the way, I chose not to jump off the bridge but to continue walking in search of help. Once there, I was received but not helped further. The next day, my psychologist gave me the contact details of a psychiatrist, and I was able to attend a first consultation shortly afterwards. I couldn't imagine going to a psychiatrist. I had suggested it to my GP a few years earlier, but he had dismissed it. He didn't think the seriousness of my problems was great enough, and with medication and conversations with the psychologist, I would manage. With that fixed idea, I crossed the threshold that day and rang the doorbell with trembling knees. I briefly told my story. For the first time, I felt my problems were taken seriously and listened to without judgement. Completely surprised but relieved, the conversation ended with a proposal for admission. Finally, I had the help I needed.

My husband couldn't cope with the idea that I would be admitted for fifteen weeks and would be away from home again a lot. Underlying this was his main message: Who will look after me now? At weekends, out of guilt, I did my best to keep the household in order and be there for him as much as possible. It hadn't dawned on me that I didn't have to care anymore but needed to be cared for. Lockdown during the coronavirus crisis was a blessing in a way because I stayed in the clinic uninterrupted for several months and was thus protected from my demanding and sexually coercive husband. I could focus on myself and concentrate all my attention on my recovery. Of course, the relationship with my husband deteriorated further because of the distance, but also from my side because the realisation of the abuse was increasingly dawning on me. A separation had been looming over the relationship for a long time, and it became a fact after the lockdown.

The initial fifteen weeks of admission ultimately turned into three years, with periods of (intermittent) discharge. It was an incredibly long and, at times, an extremely frustrating, hopeless and unrealistically arduous journey. The desire to die was very present. It always felt like I was in a pitch-black room without doors, where only a little light came through a small crack. I had to cling to that because there is no life without hope. During that time, I made a couple of attempts to end my life. The pain and suffering were unbearable at times, making death seem like bliss. And yet, time and again, I saw the light through that crack and lived on the slight hope that remained. The therapies were intense, but the bond with the therapists made me feel supported. Group therapy allowed me to slowly shed my mask of trying to appear well. Patients who were further along in their process spoke openly and without hesitation. That was quite shocking at first but gradually believable. I realised that we were all in the same boat. No one was better or worse than anyone else. Human suffering knows no status or order. In retrospect, I consider the long admission and therapy process very valuable and am very grateful for it. My self-awareness has increased (a never-ending process, by the way). I can better analyse certain situations, allowing me to better cope with myself, the world around me, and life in general, from self-destruction to self-care. I have become much more confident in myself, and I can be genuinely proud of what I have achieved and can do again at times. However, I am sometimes thrown back into depressive feelings and anxieties. This clarifies that it is continuous work and that I am not 'there' yet. The two therapy sessions a week are therefore necessary, and it is an acceptance that I will always remain mentally vulnerable. However, I am better equipped and can intervene more quickly when things go wrong.

Meanwhile, I am creating dance performances again, which is against my expectations. I had quietly put my art aside during that dark period. I didn't think it possible to return. But still, my passion for dance is so great that the urge to create has again taken over. I thoroughly enjoy being in a creative process again and being on stage. It brings me great joy and zest for life. It's coming home to my body, letting everything flow and speak in a language I've known and loved since childhood. Even the entire journey of the past few years is an inexhaustible source of inspiration.

7 C.V.D.V.

From a young age, I've struggled with anxiety. At school, it was mainly a fear of failure. I got good grades but was always terrified of not doing well. I couldn't finish my higher education; I dropped out due to overwhelming anxiety and started working. After a problematic seven-year relationship (with a narcissist), I finally found the strength to leave. I met my current partner, we bought a house, got married, and a few years later I became pregnant. Those were wonderful years, relatively anxiety free, a time of security and safety. Then, during my pregnancy (which coincided with the coronavirus pandemic), things started to go wrong due to a combination of factors. I started experiencing severe panic attacks, several a day. I couldn't function, I couldn't work, I could do nothing. Everything seemed insurmountable.

After giving birth to our daughter, I didn't immediately feel the maternal instinct. It felt like I wasn't her mother. This was also linked to my mental state at the time. I couldn't care for our daughter. My parents were with me every day, even after the birth, caring for me, our daughter and everything else because I was incapable. We tried outpatient treatment for eight months, but it wasn't successful. So, I decided to seek inpatient treatment.

A lot was discussed about my childhood and my parents. I'm an only child, and I've always felt I had a warm, protective upbringing. I had to learn to talk about my parents. I think they always did so much for me. I had never said a bad word about them, and talking about things that hadn't gone so well – not necessarily intentionally on their part – was incredibly difficult. Attributing anything to my upbringing, to 'them', felt wrong. Something inside me made me feel so guilty if I said anything negative about my parents. It became clear that my mother was dominant in my upbringing. She thinks in very black-and-white terms – it's either good or bad. Her reactions can sometimes be harsh. It's also unpredictable what reaction you'll get. This was just reality; I never questioned it; it was expected.

One day (quite late into my therapy), I said, 'You know, it feels like there's a little voice in my head constantly feeding me insecurities and anxieties.' And it wasn't me but someone else, and I gave the voice a name: Petunia, an external 'person' inside me. Why I chose that name, I don't know, but it wasn't a sweet name because the voice wasn't kind to me. I didn't consciously think about it being a female voice, but that's how it felt. It became clear that Petunia was present in everything I did, thought and undertook. Like a devil on my shoulder, a strict referee always makes me waver and doubt, presenting the worst-case scenario as the realistic outcome of my actions. I couldn't say or do anything without Petunia attaching a negative thought and an excessively negative consequence; it was either a good or a red card; there was no middle ground. I was kept small by this voice. I realised I was still behaving like the inferior one in relationships, like a child, even though I'm almost forty. That's not how I felt, but I always felt more petite than the other person, like the child in a parent-child dynamic. You have to listen to what the other person says. You have to be good and follow the rules. Otherwise, there's punishment; the other person will be angry with me. Subconsciously, I also behaved like a small child. Whenever anything happened, I'd go to my parents first, not my husband. It became clear I was still seeking my mother and father's approval – Petunia's approval? I think this also contributed to the problematic start after our daughter's birth. I was still a 'child'. I couldn't handle the responsibility or the care of another person. I'd always been able to rely on my parents, who took care of everything and protected me from everything. I was always cared for. And that's what they did in our daughter's first year of life, especially for me.

How long has Petunia been in my head? Has she been there since childhood? Has she influenced my life for so long? Did she prevent me from developing beyond childhood into an independent self, a woman, a partner, a mother? These questions surfaced. Gradually, the realisation dawned that I'd always adhered to Petunia's standards, the voice I created as a child that never disappeared. It became clear that Petunia was, in a way, an internalisation of my mother, a constantly present supervisor.

I constantly adapted; I didn't dare express my opinion; I didn't dare break the rules. Rebellion is regular in adolescence, but I didn't dare. Even in my adult life, everything had to be 'perfect' at work. But I don't measure up; I can never meet Petunia's demands. And I always want to meet those demands so much. Everyone 'must' like me, find me likeable. There's a 'need to be loved'. There's a great fear of rejection. I find that very difficult to cope with.

In my therapy, I'm now trying to detach myself from Petunia and live more according to my values and beliefs. That's not always easy. It's a search for who I am and a little frightening when I'm 'alone', wondering what I should do. Will I manage without Petunia? I'm also working on my relationship with my parents, creating more distance and finding a healthy balance. That's not easy, not for me, not for them. Ultimately, you're changing a relationship that's been formed since birth and hasn't adapted according to normal development. When they say it's difficult for them, I try to find a balance.

However, sometimes it feels difficult for me without their sounding board, but I have to try to regulate that myself. And that's sometimes hard. I'm fortunate that I can always share my thoughts with my husband. He can help me dissect my thoughts and ensure they don't feel as charged as they sometimes do in my head. I've shifted my focus from my parental home to my family. I'll talk to my husband first about what's on my mind instead of going to my parents. My family is the most important thing; that's where I find my happiness now.

Some things I can shake off better now, but others are harder. Even putting this testimony into words is very difficult. It's an amplified confrontation with what's going on in your head every day. It's very confronting. It highlights once again the 'power' Petunia has over me. That does frighten me. I want to be myself, without restrictions, without fear. I've also made enormous strides in my relationship with our daughter. Gradually, I was able to take on more and more care and responsibility for her. Our bond has improved so much; we do fun things together and enjoy each other's company. I'd do anything for her. But I realise I have to be careful not to do the same thing my parents did for me: wanting to protect her from everything. My therapy has made me very aware of how we raise her.

It remains a struggle with Petunia to this day, but I'm getting better at pushing her aside, offering resistance, saying: I am who I am, that people know who I am, and that I never act with bad intentions. If there's something others disagree with me on, then so be it. I must learn that my feelings and ideas aren't everyone's feelings. But it's perfectly okay to have my feelings. Ultimately, we are all different and unique. Not everyone fits with your personality, and that's okay. Not everyone has to like you or approve of you. Even those closest to you don't always have to agree. You can only live according to the values and norms you hold. The self-confidence to openly express and stand up for that is something I strongly aspire to. It's a process I'll be involved in for a while, but that's okay.

8 D.S.

This story begins when I'm in my early twenties, fresh out of university and starting my first job. I immediately secured a permanent contract and, with a nervous heart, I was ready to prove to myself and everyone else that I was worthwhile. Unfortunately, it became a real struggle as my past wouldn't let go. Unconsciously, my brother still held the reins. Even though I had no contact with him, I remained his puppet, constantly and unknowingly. He controlled my feelings and thoughts. I'd swallowed him whole; he was ingrained in my personality. His destructive words had become my everyday thoughts. He reappeared, distorted, in my dreams at night and directed my actions during the day. My past and present were interwoven.

My relationship with my parents was complex. Despite my cries for help then, my brother was put on a pedestal and given free rein. Because of this, I took the blame and suffered in shame. This was my fate, my just deserts. Without malice, my parents didn't do what they should have done and did what they shouldn't have. My parents were physically present (usually in a different room), and I lacked nothing material. They didn't deliberately hurt me. So, what could I possibly complain about? I felt I shouldn't complain.

I viewed the world through the eyes of the person my family said I was and should be. I thought I was myself, but I had hardly any contact with my body and individuality. I 'functioned'. Concentrating became increasingly difficult, and my memory was very selective. My thinking was slow; I absorbed little and learned slowly, like a tardy computer doing a lot unseen in the background.

Socially, I built protective walls around myself and wasn't approachable. Relaxation, peace, safety and self-confidence were (physically) alien to me. I had many physical ailments, chronic inflammations and much unexplained pain, an insatiable pain. Despite this, I didn't feel depressed or anxious and attributed these symptoms and pains to anything but emotional suffering. I enjoyed big and small things, mainly my partner and dog, and being outdoors and active. I was the patient who went to doctors with unexplained physical complaints and resolutely ticked 'no' to the question of whether I was anxious.

However, it didn't stop at physical pain and some uncertainty. Due to strange symptoms, a difficult-to-swallow comment at work and an incorrect medical diagnosis, I was forced to take sick leave. I ended up in significant uncertainty and isolation. I was offered all sorts of diagnoses and treatments, and, in the long run, the pills made me sicker rather than better. I felt abandoned, anxious and let down. I was exhausted, but it wasn't a classic depression. Contact with my in-laws was problematic. Due to the lack of acknowledgement from my parents, I decided to cut contact with my family. However, distancing myself from an unhealthy past (without a solid foundation) proved impossible. There was anything but distance; 'you can check out any time, but you can never leave'.

Eventually, I ended up in a psychiatric emergency room. I felt incredibly trapped. I panicked and, therefore, refused admission. I opted for twelve weeks of psychotherapeutic treatment in a day hospital. This got me a little further so that after a year-and-a-half of sick leave, I could gradually resume work. Fundamentally, nothing had changed, so I continued to struggle. When the bucket finally overflowed about two years later, a second treatment followed in the same day hospital. To no avail because then nothing or nobody could get through to me. Cut off from myself and others and burdened with constant suicidal thoughts, a residential admission to a clinical psychotherapeutic ward of a psychiatric hospital followed. I felt like I was going to be doing my 'life sentence' in 'prison'. It felt hopeless and certainly not a solution.

I had no trust in this admission or the people working there. Not in myself, others, society … I saw no improvement in myself, although I still wanted to give it a chance. I occasionally enjoyed certain things, but I couldn't bear the burden weighing ever more heavily on me. I couldn't correctly name what was wrong, let alone solve it. I could hardly say anything good or positive about myself and felt like an incredibly hopeless case. I was humiliated, and my courage sank into my shoes.

The first week, I was more outside the treatment walls of the psychiatric hospital than inside, and I called my partner and psychologist almost daily in disbelief. I didn't know what I was doing on the ward. I had little trust, was bitter and wasn't there to make friends. So, I didn't exactly behave sympathetically or accessibly. I clashed with rules whose purpose I didn't understand, and which seemed designed to make everything even more difficult. I was blunt and defensive, found it difficult to connect, and constantly wanted to go home, but once home, I also wanted to leave again.

I flitted from one room to another without daring to settle. I felt unsafe without being able to name it, and I fled home at the slightest confrontation. However, the insecurity was within me, so after refuelling, I quickly returned. I felt out of place, compared myself to my fellow patients and thought I had no traumas to discuss. I must admit that I had problems with – you'll never guess – *myself.*

It took me time to talk, keep repeating myself, and hear myself go on ad nauseam. To find a place among a mass of people with difficulties in a system with many rules. Also, I needed to form attachments for the first time. This was something I strongly resisted because who wants to get attached to a psychiatric hospital, I thought. That seemed like digging your own grave. It took a long time to connect with patients and staff. I was constantly misunderstood because I couldn't explain myself enough or came across wrong. I felt I couldn't turn to anyone. I had difficulty with my psychologist at the time, with the psychiatrist ... I made friends but also regularly got into conflict.

I cried, laughed, sang, shouted ... on the ward, and felt a whole arsenal of emotions and feelings. I went through many processes. For example, from walking around the nurses' station in a wide arc to being drawn to their blue armchairs. Often not fully understanding why at the time and with much resistance. In retrospect, they were all useful 'phases'; I'm glad they happened and are now behind me. The less I wondered what I was doing, where it was all leading and whether it would improve me, the more confidence I gained and the smoother my progress became. Eventually, I increasingly understood what clinical psychotherapy was doing to me and that every daily confrontation had a direct link to my past. Psychotherapy doesn't cure; it mainly brings meaning.

I started with a full admission to participate, but I needed the security to 'escape' home if it became unbearable. This happened quite frequently at the beginning and was also necessary to persevere. After that, I moved on to day therapy. Tailored to my needs, day therapy and full admission alternated. We worked towards completion by moving to combined day therapy with a new job (gradual return to work). The job proved to be very disappointing. I had already gained some insights, but there wasn't enough lived-through knowledge or sufficient foundation to be resilient. Therefore, letting go of the psychiatric hospital didn't work either.

On the advice of the ward, I stopped the job and returned to full admission. The disappointment and panic were enormous, and I felt worse than ever. I had to go through a severe suicidal phase. Therapy did little because of my clouded thinking, and the pills gave me a frighteningly immobilising feeling. I felt more hopeless than ever. I ended up in a different living group, better suited to the current process, but where I could count on little understanding from my fellow patients. I thought I had already reached the bottom of the pit, but there was still a cellar. Against all advice, I decided to go on a ten-day trip with my partner. Our sporty and adventurous trips have always been a blessing, and it worked this time, too: nature, freedom, togetherness and lots of exercise blew some of the dark mist out of my head.

Once back, I started again with a full admission. To my surprise, I came up with new themes. I went through the same process of full admission to day therapy to combined day therapy at an accelerated pace. I felt how my attachment had changed. However unusual this felt, I let it happen. I found a new job and held onto the ward for a while via an aftercare programme (half a day per week). The job turned out to be safer than the previous one but, intellectually, it was so far below my level that it didn't do me any good. Then, too, I had to drop out again, but it all went without much turbulence this time. My professional situation remained unstable for a long time, but I stayed afloat and felt surrounded and supported for the first time.

My psychotherapeutic process took the necessary time, and that proved to be required. In terms of duration, I had a period of weeks in mind, but it became years. If I had known at the outset that this would be such a complex and lengthy process, I would never have started it. Yet I'm glad I persevered and took my time; I needed the long duration of my admissions, and what else would I have done? The break between the two admissions was necessary to feel and see where things were still not going well.

It was touch and go. If I hadn't bonded with specific caregivers during my first admission, I might have given up at the start of the second. Although therapy couldn't provide me with all my needs, I'm glad I didn't drop out or deviate. That would not have done me any good regarding trust and attachment.

Now I realise that you only know what 'insecurity' is once you know 'safety'. The first step in my process was acknowledging and understanding. Only much later did compassion, gentleness and self-worth come for the first time. I am increasingly connecting with myself, with more expression and balance and fewer question marks, confusion and exaggerations. I have become less withdrawn. Everything built up remains fragile, but stability steadily grows through trial and error. Only now is my potential emerging, and I stand on my own two feet with a small basis of self-confidence and trust. Setbacks no longer completely knock me down, as I have finally acquired a foundation; it's something invisible but essential for coping with life. Something that only strikes me after the storm, which means that the 'what if' anxiety remains somewhat palpable.

My body is still complex; the body keeps the score. It seems still dysregulated and can still take over my emotions when they are unbearable or don't want to be felt. Sometimes, this is a precise observation. Sometimes, it happens to me, and it's guesswork about cause and solution. What I currently find most challenging to cope with is the feeling of being at the mercy of a problematic body and having to rely on others. This immediately evokes an (old) feeling of dependence and loss of control. I don't get rid of my extreme sobriety, antennae and distrust of others, but somewhere, I don't want to either. I flourish when I feel I have control over my emotions and body. I fear that the problematic relationship with my own body will remain like this for a while, but I am hopeful because I see positive progress.

Emotionally, I am probably confronted with my past daily, but not as before. An old wound is easily touched, but without me acting on it. The confrontations happen in a very conscious way. The link is immediately apparent; the emotion is often quickly felt and can be expressed in words. It continues to affect me, and I would also be heartless towards myself if it weren't so. I have a history and am more complex at these moments. Realising that I have a backlog compared to others evokes anger and compassion. At other times, my history can be my strength. This ultimately also brought a clear advantage in the workplace: it makes me an empathetic, feeling and sensitive being, as well as a self-aware helper with an extra sense.

Clinical psychotherapy helped me not only to connect with myself but also with others. It works on a deeper level, something that had never been possible for me in outpatient therapy.

I am happy with the friends and hobbies I now have. I have better contact with my parents again (as far as possible). I have now been together with the best and dearest partner in the world for twelve years. Our relationship has become stronger and more stable, and we are gradually becoming more 'equal' partners. I can now make choices like getting married and renovating with a more peaceful heart. I know better who I am and what I want. I have some more reserve and a small base to fall back on. There are still ups and downs, but I must face life again. I can now confidently be 'a live wire' again. I still have weekly psychotherapy. The conversations are to the point and cover the persistent difficult things and the sound/new things that bring about all sorts of consequences. My past is effectively becoming my past. It predicts my future less and less. I'm not finished yet, but I'm hopeful, given the path I've already travelled.

9 D.V.

It's difficult to trace back to the start of my psychotherapy; for me, it equates to the beginning of psychoanalytic therapy. Writing about that initial period, where a 'not-knowing' defined everything, from the perspective of today's 'knowledge' is challenging. I'll try to place myself back in that time, but that 'knowing' will inevitably intrude.

My experience with therapy began very early. In primary school, I was bullied, or at least that's how I perceived it. I was called a faggot or a sissy, although I didn't even know what these words meant at the time. I asked my mother, and she explained that it was a derogatory term for a gay man, pointing out the only openly 'effeminate' gay man in the village as an example. I was a frightened little boy who couldn't leave his mother at the school gates, but perhaps it was (also) the other way around. The other children saw this and made fun of me. My parents contacted a child psychiatrist they had previously seen for my brother. That wasn't a positive experience. I remember I was about eleven, having to draw a castle and its defences. I drew a castle and little sticks to prevent the castle from being attacked. The child psychiatrist said it was nice, all those little plants, but that it needed to be a defence. I didn't understand; they didn't even ask me what I'd drawn. The conclusion was that I had a motor disorder. I had to undergo physiotherapy because my motor skills weren't where they should have been for my age.

For years, I underwent therapy with a physiotherapist who was supposed to make me less clumsy and stop me from moving like a 'Jeanette'. Even now, on a dance floor, that stiff posture remains despite all the therapy. My father was advised to continue teasing me so I would toughen up. Later, I realised it was a form of goading. I see him doing it with his grandchildren now. I felt abandoned.

During puberty, I realised I had feelings for other boys. As always, my mother was my first refuge. That felt very heavy and constricted, partly due to my Catholic upbringing. My parents returned to the child psychiatrist, who noted that I could talk well to my mother and didn't think further therapy was necessary. In retrospect, she pushed me under my mother's wing, a place I desperately wanted to escape from but lacked the strength to do so. My mother had, in effect, given me the message in childhood that the whole world was unsafe and that I should seek safety with her. That evening, I had suicidal thoughts for the first time.

Later, in my teens – I would have been about sixteen – I started contextual therapy at the General Welfare Centre. I felt an unease I couldn't explain, partly caused by my burgeoning homosexual feelings, but mainly, and I can say this in hindsight, because it was time to stand on my own two feet and leave the parental nest. I don't have negative memories of this therapy. I could be myself and talk, but it didn't achieve much. Attempts to leave home failed.

I started psychoanalysis when my situation became acute. I went to university and lived in halls, but after graduating as a social worker, it was time to face the world. I started experiencing panic attacks. I endlessly worried about whether or not I had homosexual feelings. Was I a Jeanette? I struggled to set boundaries in homosexual relationships, feeling confused and unhappy.

It was utter chaos. I also suffered from anger outbursts, self-harm and periods of excessive drinking.

Initially, I was admitted to a psychotherapeutic centre for three months. Psychoanalysis didn't appeal to me at the time, and after discharge, I tried behavioural therapy. The outpatient behavioural therapy transitioned into day therapy. It was a challenging period that, in retrospect, felt like being in 'a detention centre'. Nothing happened; it was a period of complete stagnation. Finding the proper psychotherapy proved far from straightforward. Finding appropriate care, support and psychotherapy was a truly (desperate) search. After a suicide attempt, I ended up in a psychiatric intensive care unit. From there, I was referred to a clinical psychotherapeutic ward. In hindsight, that's where therapy truly began.

At that point, I expected a three-month admission, after which everything would be resolved. Ultimately, after a relatively extended residential stay, it turned out to be a process spanning several years, with periods of inpatient and day therapy alternating. At the same time, I began outpatient psychoanalysis. This was twenty years ago; except for a week's 'rest', I haven't been admitted to a psychiatric ward since.

My therapy consisted of two sessions a week with my psychoanalyst and what was called 'process guidance' roughly every six to eight weeks. Currently, since my 'separation', I still have one weekly session with my psychoanalyst; the process guidance has naturally faded away.

Once admitted to a psychiatric ward, I felt listened to for the first time. Everything was questioned and explored; there were no taboos. There was no advice, rules to follow, or tasks to complete … My symptom of an 'irresistible urge' for homosexual contact was often treated with the advice to simply accept that I was homosexual. Previous therapies quickly dismissed the burden I felt from constantly seeking and hunting for sexual contact. Now, the underlying reasons for this impulsive behaviour were explored. What was my childhood like? What was my relationship with my parents? How was I raised? … It was the start of a journey of self-discovery.

My sexual orientation was also questioned. Early in my admission, I began a heterosexual relationship that lasted seventeen years. I also became a father through adoption. This relationship has ended, and I am entirely alone for the first time. In a way, this brings me back to the starting point of my therapy. The anxiety that was there then has returned. Still, now I know that's what it's fundamentally about: being overprotected, with an overly present, anxious mother and an absent father who was goading when he was around. My ex-partner continued that role.

As I became increasingly independent and assertive under the influence of therapy, the relationship ceased to work. So the work is still not finished. I continue to analyse how this new situation affects me and why it frightens me. For the first time in my life, I am truly alone. I moved from one symbiotic relationship (with my mother) into another (with my ex-partner). In the meantime, I have chosen to live my life as a gay man but, at the moment, I am a single father with a six-year-old son. My best friend often tells me I'm a Jeanette, and you know what? I don't care anymore. The burden and negativity associated with that word have entirely disappeared. I sometimes use the word myself. Because besides therapy, the situation you find yourself in is also crucial, at least for me.

When my ex and I tried to conceive through insemination and IVF (in vitro fertilisation) treatments, it only made my struggle with my 'masculinity' more difficult. The 'separation', in turn, revealed other things. Becoming a father allowed me to leave behind the incredible anger that the journey in therapy produced. I could see that my parents were just people who had made many mistakes. I also didn't have everything figured out when I became a father. Therapy and the search for the 'why' made me very angry with my parents. What mistakes my parents had made!

The 'irresistible urge' is under control; it was a mechanism, I now know, to vent my anger ('fuck!'). However strange it may sound, I have had fewer homosexual encounters than during my relationship. My ex-partner made me so angry that they could drive me into a corner.

The changes are too numerous to mention; I am a completely different person than when I started therapy. Through my therapeutic process, I developed a personality that wasn't there before. I have become someone. I have become assertive; I give my opinion. I have a responsible job. I work daily with vulnerable people, and twenty years ago, I could have been on the same side as the staff I now work with. I would never have thought this possible; I manage and supervise about fifteen employees. The way I interact with the 'target group' is very much shaped by the therapy I underwent and still undergo. That small, vulnerable bird I once was has largely disappeared. I stand my ground. Before this, I also ran my own business for seven years.

For example, I struggled a lot with the question of whether I was a (real) man; I also associated homosexuality with 'not being a man'. Now, this is no longer an issue for me. I discovered and learned that being male and female is not a given. I recently read a quote from someone who wrote: 'Gender is the first fact in life and simultaneously the first illusion.' I have shaped myself as a man, a self-made man. I feel masculine, and all the insecurity that used to go with it has disappeared. That's sometimes the strange thing about my therapeutic process: suddenly, a symptom, a problem, an issue ... disappears without anything being done about it.

However, life is still a learning process, and I don't plan to stop the therapy I'm undergoing. The work is not yet finished, and perhaps it never will be, which doesn't mean therapy will remain necessary until the end of my days. This applies to many people, if not all people; we are constantly evolving. Recently, I received a compliment from a good friend: 'I don't know anyone who knows themselves as well as you do.' I think it's also true that I know myself very well and notice processes and blind spots ... in others faster than the average person. I don't shy away from them, neither in myself nor in others. That leads to depth. That has allowed me to develop a very 'rich' life with only a few friends but intense friendships.

I do notice that when I have a date with a man with a view to a relationship, it sometimes clashes with the fact that I see they don't know themselves. I am also a father in a different way than my father was. I can question myself, perhaps too much sometimes. My fatherhood remains my weak point; I want to do it well. I'm doing quite well. I am aware of the impact of upbringing on a child's later life, my child's life.

All this and numerous other changes are mainly attributable to my years of therapy. What strikes me is that the expectations I had at the beginning of my therapeutic process are different from the provisional 'result'. I expected to fix things quickly but gradually discovered that the foundation laid in my childhood was flawed.

It was a process of trial and error – talking, talking and talking again. Repeating and repeating, often the same things, and my therapist's small, usually short but insightful interventions. A thought-provoking question. A comment that sometimes hits the mark perfectly … In this way, I grew, developed a vision, gained self-knowledge, learned to deal with certain situations differently … The intensity of a twice-weekly therapeutic session meant that no detail was overlooked. Everything I experienced was discussed.

In therapy, I sometimes miss a pat on the back, confirmation, advice … At the same time, I understand that this could have led to yet another 'present' mother in my life. Because of that, I experienced my psychoanalyst as somewhat cold but very professional.

As for the 'process supervision', this has always been a valuable addition to viewing things from a distance and having them considered by someone else. The need for this is now less (or no longer) present than it was a year ago. The process supervision was sometimes shocking, as I am pretty 'sensitive', but ultimately it led to new insights, or to insights that I initially disregarded. The fact that a man carried out this supervision process did bring a certain balance to the therapeutic process. I also underwent an evolution within that process of supervision. I was afraid of the supervisor and accepted everything he said as accurate. I had not known that in my life, a male figure. Eventually, I went to the process supervision without fear and could disagree with the insights given.

This evolution, this process, has ultimately been an essential part of 'making myself' without wanting to suggest that 'myself' is a fixed fact, an unshakeable and unchanging given. Therapy has taught me that movement and change … are possible and that nothing needs to be fixed in advance, but everything can be questioned. This previously led to significant uncertainty; now, it leads to a feeling of incredible freedom.

Previously, I was guided by the dominant mother within me and the absent father who made me yearn to fill this void. Through the therapeutic process, I have gained a great deal of freedom. The freedom to choose who I want to become and do what I want is no longer driven by an invisible force called the unconscious. The therapeutic process can be summarised as analysing, becoming aware, and acting accordingly.

10 D.V.D.C.

For years, I had lived on the edge, pushing myself so far that my body finally said: Stop! This was both a literal and a figurative stop. I experienced severe anxiety and panic attacks that caused me to lose control of my body. I started shaking and trembling and lost touch with reality. It was as if my life suddenly came to a standstill, trapped in a dark circle of fear and despair from which I could find no escape.

Before I started my current therapy, I had already tried different forms of help. For example, I had already undergone cognitive behavioural therapy, but this didn't help me. I also tried medication in various forms in a desperate search for something that could rescue me from this hell. In addition, I visited a sleep clinic because I had hardly slept for years. Stress, anxiety, nightmares, insomnia, depressive and hyper episodes dominated my life. When I received a phone call saying I could be admitted to the Attachment and Trauma ward, I didn't know what to expect. I was scared but also relieved. On the one hand, it felt like a wonderful birthday present; I finally hoped to find some peace somewhere, a feeling of safety and stability. This was my very first admission after years of traumatic experiences.

My psychotherapist was an extraordinary woman. For the first time, I dared to tell her everything. It did take a while before I dared to let go of the darkest details, but gradually, she won my trust. We had an excellent connection and, based on that, I could lower my walls progressively. This safe space enabled me to be open about my feelings and experiences, something I had never been able to do before.

The psychotherapy itself took some getting used to. It was mainly a lot of talking and reflecting on how everything had come about. For years, I had lived with the idea that it was all my fault, but eventually, I began to see that I was far too young to have experienced so many negative experiences without help from my parents. Reflecting on my parent role, I realised I would never treat my child similarly. These insights were confronting but also liberating. By repeating the events many times, I eventually saw that it wasn't my fault. The group sessions confirmed that I wasn't alone. It was a relief to discover that others had similar experiences and feelings. This feeling of shared knowledge and understanding gave me strength.

What helped me most was the feeling of being safe somewhere. It was a relief to hear that my anxiety and panic attacks were understandable after everything I had been through. I no longer had to walk on eggshells. The idea that someone was listening to me was essential to my process. The difficult conversation with my mother, in which I finally got clarity about my attachment issues, was also an important step. With the support of my psychotherapist and contextual therapist, we were able to have this conversation, and I am still very grateful for that.

I can't say there was anything that didn't help me. Every session, big or small, has added value to my life. Every step, however tricky, brought me closer to my recovery. To this day, my process is still ongoing. I was admitted for a year, and it remains a constant challenge to work on yourself and learn to understand yourself, both physically and emotionally. In the first week, I was in complete admission because I was utterly in survival mode. Then, I followed the regular full admission, where I could go home at weekends and Wednesday afternoons. Sometimes, I could stay a few nights for a safety net when it was difficult. I still miss that safe place with the 'mother clinic' sometimes. Now, I'm doing outpatient therapy, which is more challenging because you have to put everything into practice outside the hospital.

I have learned to accept myself for who I am and to embrace my anxiety and panic attacks, making them less severe. I have learned safety and a warm nest where there is trust. This has given my life a new direction. I have gained a new perspective on life and found recognition for my experiences. The feeling of safety and no longer being put down for the slightest things has given me so much. It was more than worth it.

My evolution is terrific, especially in how I look at my children. What you haven't learned, you can never pass on or use. My anxiety and panic attacks have been minimised, and if I have one, I accept it as usual. The tools I have been given to use in real life and recognising my signals when they become too much are invaluable. My admission was one of the best gifts in my life. It wasn't very easy, but I am proud that I did it. Also, thank you for all the support and love from the admission, the wonderful people, and the friendships developed at the clinic. It was more than worth it. I can live again! This story describes my journey from despair to recovery. It shows the importance of getting the right help, learning to see your worth, and understanding that you are not alone. It is a story of hope and healing, a testament to therapy's power and finding your way to a better life.

11 E.G.

It was the question of whether what I was feeling was justified that led me to psychotherapy. I wanted acknowledgement of my pain and, at the same time, to delve deeper and finally understand why life feels like survival for me. What is the cause of my anxieties and frustrations? Why am I so often insecure? Where does this constant self-doubt come from? Why am I unhappy when I have everything to be happy?

For a long time, I had been asking myself questions for which I had never found a satisfactory answer in the well-trodden paths or the superficial/short-term solutions. Questions I was good at hiding … until a child was born, and

I was subsequently presented with one mirror after another. This led to immense friction, insomnia, even more depressive moods and stress-related issues that spread like wildfire through my life (and that of my family). It was when I could escape no more demons and my days turned pitch black that I took a step towards psychotherapy. A path I had never planned for myself and, somehow, it felt like a confirmation of my failure. But I was at a dead end; I saw no way out; even losing myself in another professional project (my *modus vivendi* when faced with problems) was no longer an option as I was physically drained. I had no choice but to admit that the answer didn't lie in another goal but in stopping and looking at what was holding me back. I wanted to understand. And I couldn't do that alone; I'd tried for thirty-five years. It was the first time I had asked for professional help. Something I found incredibly difficult, but I knew it was now or never.

The decision to work with my psychiatrist wasn't entirely rational. It was a combination of connecting with his books and the fact that I could start therapy very quickly, which instantly gave me a feeling of validation: my pain wasn't imagined. Because somewhere, I still considered myself a great drama queen with no reason or time to be preoccupied with self-centred life questions. But the psychiatrist legitimised my concerns; he listened and didn't dismiss anything, however much I tried to do so. What followed was a painful but highly instructive six-month journey, with a weekly session on Wednesdays.

I was familiar with the Freudian school through my psychology training. Still, it wasn't until I was lying on the couch myself that I truly understood what a psychotherapeutic process entails. And how raw and brutal it is. Haltingly, I tried to articulate as clearly as possible what I felt and where I thought things were going wrong. I had thought about it for so long, yet I sometimes seemed to have run out of things to say and found myself at a dead end. Then I would fall silent, sometimes for minutes; it felt like my mind was locked. Through his questioning, he made me reflect on my insights. On all the frameworks I had set up, all the ideas I clung to, all the words that shaped my reality. The result was that the ground kept shifting beneath my feet, and I was further stripped down until only the harsh reality remained. The naked truth. It felt as if I was face-to-face with everything I hadn't wanted to look at until then. Or everything I hadn't been able to see is also possible.

I understood better and better why my life looked the way it did. The causes, the consequences. I became aware of my patterns and those of others. By stopping, a process of awareness had been set in motion. Everything passed in review, from traumatic events from the past that I had always minimised to conversations that had lingered for years and situations that suddenly took on a completely different aspect. The psychiatrist helped me not to get stuck in my thoughts. To keep moving forward and to look at things from a different perspective.

Rationally, I saw the bigger picture after a few months; I understood what led to what and why things were as they were, but emotionally, I was still stuck. I couldn't physically relax during psychotherapy, nor could I break down the walls around my heart. I felt an apparent disconnect between my head and my body. That was also one of my problems. And the reason I could dryly and almost on autopilot illuminate traumas on Wednesdays but then crash on Thursdays. The processing always came a day later. When I was alone, that made me realise that alongside talk therapy, I also needed other outlets to connect with (the pain in) my body. The insights I had gained from talking had to be able to translate physically as well. Because understanding is one thing, but implementing it is something else. Although they are inextricably linked, my sorrow could never have been detached if I hadn't first mentally escaped from my prison.

Yoga and meditation sessions, cold-water therapy, detoxing, acupuncture, writing ... I filled my diary with all sorts of treatments that could bring me closer to myself. Some I only managed for a short time. Others, such as breathing exercises, have become a permanent part of my life. The combination of psychotherapy with alternative emotional therapies proved to accelerate my healing. However, it was excruciating to feel life finally and my past. Everything came loose. During that same period, I discovered lumps in my breast. Then, I had to choose where my energy and focus were most urgently needed. That's why I stopped psychotherapy and devoted myself entirely to my physical recovery.

What became clear to me in this therapy is how much you are at the wheel yourself. How much control do you retain, and are you forced into? This is tricky because you want to be rescued when life slips through your fingers and only questions remain. But psychoanalysis taught me that no one can rescue me except myself. That the answer lies nowhere except within me. In the long run, it resulted in an immensely liberating and empowering feeling. At first, it confused me how empathetic yet also very clearly defined my psychiatrist was. How sessions could end abruptly when time was up, for example. Then I was suddenly outside again, back on my own, with a head full of new realisations. Because with that freedom came responsibility. I was going to have to do it myself.

Personal input and strong motivation are crucial in this therapy. It doesn't stop after the session; that's when it begins. Keeping a diary in which I wrote down our conversations and the insights that arose from them proved to be an essential part of seeing my progress. Because when you're in the middle of a process, it doesn't seem that way. Yet it was remarkable how thoughts could shift in just a few weeks because the psychiatrist kept the ball rolling. That gave me an immense boost to know that everything I was going through actually led to something, that real change was taking place and that I was indeed going in the right direction.

Looking back, such intensive treatment was exactly what I needed to learn to stand on my own two feet, form my conclusions, and acknowledge and speak my truth. After a lifetime of following and bending, it was a relief that someone didn't tell me what to do but let me be. It directly and indirectly reminded me that I can do this (by myself). My hand wasn't held but, in a way, I didn't want that either.

The fact that I stopped my therapy myself was, for me, another confirmation that I was starting to take my steps. I also knew that I could go back; the psychiatrist had assured me of that. But however dark the reality, however much everything was falling apart, I gained confidence in myself, and that's what had always been missing.

It's impossible to pinpoint the exact moment when I was cured; where is the line between being ill and being healthy anyway? Who decides that? Someone else or me? Are you ever cured? Was I sick ever, or is this simply part of life? It concretely means that I no longer feel the backpack on my shoulders. I still see it there; it's beside me but no longer holds me back. On the contrary, it has become invaluable in knowing what choices I should and should not make, what is essential in life, how important it is to be yourself ... and the realisation that everyone has their backpack. All in all, it took a good two years, including the six months of psychoanalysis, to finally let go of the soul pain and accompanying stress. I've slept through the night for the first time, which is a good sign.

I can only be grateful for the standstill because it obliged me to think about things I wasn't even aware of but which were governing my life. During a session with the psychiatrist, I once compared myself to a tree, how my proud oak had first become a weeping willow, then a pollarded willow, and how, eventually, my branches had been completely broken. My tree eventually died, but my roots are alive as never before. I am grateful that I can now shape my form.

12 E.R.C.

Summer 2014. What should have been a fantastic family moment turned out entirely differently. A week after the birth of our eldest daughter, I experienced postpartum psychosis. I had never experienced mental health problems before. I was in the middle of the storm at the age of twenty-seven.

My husband and I had chosen a home birth together. The moment surrounding the birth, at home in our familiar surroundings with a GP and midwife nearby, felt very comfortable and relaxed. The birth of my daughter went smoothly. I breastfed, and in retrospect this, along with the nights of less sleep, physically and ultimately mentally exhausted me. I saw connections everywhere, wanted to write everything down, was very suspicious of men ... On the evening of the crisis, I even refused to get into the car with my husband to go to the hospital. As a result, an ambulance picked me up.

The GP arranged for the mother and child to be admitted to a hospital, for which I am still very grateful. This meant that during my admission to the psychiatric ward, I could often go and see my daughter, help wash her and give her bottles. She stayed in maternity. The ability to call the nurses on the maternity ward at any time to find out how she was doing reassured me enormously. At the beginning of the psychosis and during admission to A&E (Accident and Emergency), I felt completely 'open' in my head; I was susceptible to noise, light and background conversations and had several flashbacks. Fortunately, I responded relatively quickly to the medication. I do remember the significant fatigue I was feeling. It took lots of energy to climb the stairs to maternity, wash my baby and give her a bottle. After a few weeks, we were allowed to go home.

Postnatal support and later family support provided much assistance. A daily schedule and structure were vital to me, as was getting enough rest. In the meantime, I had regular conversations with a psychotherapist who tried to explain to me what had happened. She was one of the first people I told about what had happened to me in my childhood.

I had suppressed myself for a long time and bottled everything up. When I was six, my parents separated. My mother was an alcoholic and later became depressed. The main image I remember from before I was six is the test pattern on our television in the living room and how I sat there watching it alone. It's the test pattern from the seventies with various blocks and bright colours placed in a ball. It came on screen when the programmes were over, very late at night. Mother was exhausted on the sofa, sleeping off her drunkenness, and my father wasn't home yet. Occasionally, I still see myself standing by my crying sister's cradle, trying to comfort her, or how I was listening at the top of the stairs to their arguments. Alone and quiet. A quiet, well-behaved girl, that's how others described me.

The situation only worsened after the separation. My four-years-younger sister and I were assigned to my mother. In concrete terms, we mainly lived with her and went to my father's for a weekend every two weeks; he was now living with a partner. Because of her alcoholism, depression and the medication she had to take, my mother was unable to care for us. I mainly remember the hunger, the boredom and the care I tried to take over. I tried to get my mother's attention by cooking, shopping, cleaning, making coffee and surprising her, but it was usually in vain. Many evenings in bed, I planned to run away from home. Many people in my environment didn't realise how bad the situation was. My situation improved somewhat from age fifteen because I could sometimes meet up with friends and go out. I started my higher education in halls of residence and met my husband. I graduated with a Bachelor of Nursing and then obtained a Master's.

Until my delivery, there was no time or space for grief, therapy and healing. However, the postnatal psychosis forced me to stop. After my first hospital admission and the first few months at home, during which depression also manifested itself, I decided to start a hobby for myself. I had been fascinated by tai chi for a long time and enrolled in classes. This was the start of a lifelong passion that would teach me a great deal: through the exercises, I learned to feel my body and quiet my mind; I learned to relax more deeply and became more aware of myself, my behaviour and how I reacted to my environment. Tai chi gave me much strength at times when things were going downhill for me and I was struggling with dark thoughts, for example. The lessons, exercises and meditation gave me hope and perseverance.

That one postnatal psychosis was, unfortunately, not the last, no, despite taking antipsychotics and antidepressants and outpatient follow-up with a psychiatrist and psychologist, several other admissions followed (I've somewhat lost count), each time requiring admission. The psychoses were usually triggered by periods of intense (emotional) stress, sleep deprivation or hormonal changes during my pregnancy. They usually manifested as confusion, suspicion and slowed thinking. They all started with admission to the emergency psychiatric service (EPS), where peace and quiet (except in the seclusion room) is far to seek, making it a far from ideal environment if you have a psychosis. I do remember a meaningful conversation with a night nurse at the EPS who, after an anxiety attack, said to me: 'You still have everything: you have a husband, two children, a job you love and a house. Do you realise that?' Try keeping all of that …

Moving from the busy emergency psychiatric service to a 'normal' psychiatric ward was always a relief. I particularly remember my second-to-last admission when I was six months pregnant with my youngest daughter. I was suffering from dark thoughts and eventually ended up in the seclusion room. I experienced inhumane conditions there, which I could write a whole book about. Not to mention the lack of communication with my husband. His concerns and needs as a father and husband of someone with recurrent psychoses were ignored entirely. There were no attempts in the hospital to involve, inform or include my husband in the admissions; quite the opposite – something I still regret to this day.

During my last admission for psychosis, about ten years ago, I realised that I wanted to get rid of the psychoses or avoid relapse as much as possible. In the hospital, I pressed for a transfer to a psychiatric hospital. I longed for a green environment and nature to recharge and find peace. Immediately after the admission interview, I ended up in the short-stay ward, where a nurse kindly welcomed me. On the first night, I experienced another psychosis, which meant I ended up in seclusion again. However, this seclusion room felt less threatening than the ones I knew from the general hospital.

This was because I usually saw the same nurse, who was calm and friendly and always tried to explain what would happen and what medication I was getting. I also remember fits of rage, but gradually, I became more tranquil. People cared for you; your key worker followed everything up. The approach was also totally different: the team mainly let you get to know your strengths, the possibilities you had, instead of your limitations, and the importance of self-care. Gradually, it became clear that a more prolonged admission was necessary, and I was transferred to a clinical psychotherapy unit. When I arrived on that ward, I was someone who had withdrawn into their shell, who didn't dare to speak up and certainly wouldn't voice their opinion. What was new was that I ended up in a three-person room, which was an adjustment for me. I needed silence and peace after the intense therapies I had been trying to follow. The noises in the room and never being alone were difficult for me. I found peace in walking in the park or writing in my diary. It was reassuring that I could always request a conversation with my key worker.

The therapy programmes were drawn up with my input. I followed creative therapy and cooking activities and was allowed to swim after a while. Music therapy, drama sessions and dance therapy also brought me a lot. On the piano, I gave sound to my feelings. Your feelings during those sessions spoke volumes; words were no longer necessary. Drama was gruelling, stepping outside your comfort zone, stepping into roles that mirrored people who evoked something in yourself. It's confronting and sometimes raw, but you could learn something from it. And that's why I was there, wasn't I?

During the admission, visits from my husband and children were real highlights, as were weekends at home. My eldest, now eight, participated in CPMP (children of parents with mental problems) sessions, in which they tried to explain to her what was wrong with me. The group sessions with the psychiatrist are also etched in my memory. With about eight patients, we were regularly invited to his office. We were allowed to express what had affected us or what we were dealing with. It felt like 'survival of the fittest'; the bravest, or the one whose emotions were so high, spoke up. I learned assertiveness, standing up for myself, and expressing myself powerfully and concisely. But we were always listened to; space was created for our feelings. I learned that expressing your feelings was allowed and possible.

Ultimately, my clinical psychotherapy lasted eight months, followed by about four months of first weekly and then monthly day therapy. I was discharged with regular appointments with the psychiatrist and psychologist (to this day) and a telephone number where I could reach the ward. Despite this support, I experienced the step back home as enormous: taking on the various roles again, increasing time pressure and many stimuli. This is coupled with the vast taboo that still rests on mental illness and mental resilience in our society. After all, you talk much more quickly about a broken leg than about psychosis and admission to a psychiatric hospital. During outpatient psychotherapy, I was thankfully able to vent. Initially, this was mostly about what was going wrong: difficulties, tensions and arguments ... Gradually, I also gained more insight into the trauma of my childhood, how I had become who I am now and what I could do about it. Working on myself was certainly not over after my discharge (and it never will be).

I gradually discovered myself as a compassionate, unbalanced, serious person who always exceeded her limits when caring for others. In the meantime, I know that if I respect my limits I can connect more with my body. I conserve more energy by learning to listen to my body's signals. For many years of my illness, I slept and rested a lot, even during the day, and had no more energy to do any self-care. I learned that it is imperative not to postpone even tiny things, such as a walk, a relaxing bath, breathing exercises ... By doing this self-care regularly, you gain energy; you learn to care for yourself.

Also, feeling, learning to express my feelings and asking for what I needed was a long and arduous journey. The feeling was something I had unlearned during my childhood. Allowing it would have caused too much pain at the time. During this painful realisation and processing, several meaningful people in my life inspired me about the importance of positive thinking and optimism, which we as human beings are so capable of. You know, you always have a choice. Also, my faith and trust, as well as the visits, phone calls and uplifting mail, kept me going.

After some time, I managed to resume my part-time job. My employer has continuously supported me during my illness. Continuing to work was very important to me; I learned to believe in myself again, and it gave me structure. I resumed my job initially, but there were many absences due to illness. My husband and I learned to detect the signals that precede a psychosis or depression more quickly. The GP also played an important role here; my mental health process and crises were discussed and closely monitored each time. The periods of illness became shorter, and this year I haven't had to miss a single day. I also feel better when something throws me off balance, and by taking a break more quickly and recharging in nature, exercising, cocooning at home or meeting up with friends ... I don't get so far out of balance.

For a year now, I have also been supported by a homoeopath. In my opinion, the homoeopathic support has ensured that I have been able to wean myself off the antipsychotics and antidepressants completely. Now, I can say that, after seventeen years, I have been entirely medication-free for six months. I am pleased again. I managed to combine my household with a part-time job and continue my process of self-discovery. However, I remain very aware of my vulnerability. I learned a lot and am enormously grateful for all the people who have accompanied and supported me during this journey, especially my husband, who has had much patience and unconditionally supported me during the many ups and downs of the past years. Also, my daughters, especially my eldest, often missed their mother during the admissions and absences. My future, therefore, lies primarily at home with my family, catching up on precious moments, discovering beautiful and fun things together, and being there as a mother and wife.

13 G.D.

My father was a tyrannical, narcissistic and frustrated man with a sadistic streak. My mother was a neurotic, compulsive and paranoid woman. Together, they formed a destructive couple. Domestic violence, both psychological and physical, was the order of the day. I am convinced, however, that they did their best to be good parents, or at least what they considered to be so.

Practically and materially, I was not neglected. To add to this, from what was told about me, I was not a 'typical' child and may have been more in the line of fire as a result. Growing up in 'the land of the beaten children', I did not know who or what I was when I fled the parental home through marriage at the age of twenty-one. My self-image flirted with zero. The only thing I was sure of was how it should not be. But I went full throttle for a utopian life that, with hindsight, could not exist.

Convinced that I had married the perfect woman, I lived for her and my four children. As Neeltje Maria Min puts it, 'For those I love, I will be named'. After a few years, when it became clear that my parents were continuing their destructive work in my life and that I could expect little or no support from my brothers and sisters, I broke with my family. Conflicts at home and work with my hierarchical superiors taught me that not all problems were solved that way. I felt guilty about everything that went wrong around me. In my mid-twenties, I felt utterly exhausted and constantly tired. Everything I undertook eventually went wrong, no matter how hard I tried. Suicidal thoughts emerged and even became concrete plans. I was referred to a neuropsychiatrist via my GP. After one conversation in which I felt anything but taken seriously, the diagnosis was depression, and the solution was a box of pills. It was still in the pre-Prozac era. As a result of the side effects of that medication, I felt even worse and stopped taking it soon after.

In the meantime, I regularly found release in excessive drinking. In some waiting room, I came across an article about a famous Flemish actress in which she testified about her traumatic childhood and the help she found through psychotherapy. This prompted me to start outpatient therapy with a psychologist. After a while, I stopped this again due to the high cost and the lack of tangible results. The drinking escalated and turned into a serious alcohol problem, which, of course, led to growing relationship problems. In the meantime, there was only treatment (with antidepressants) by the GP(s). Referral to specialised help was not considered necessary and even undesirable …

At some point, around the age of forty, I realised that I was in the process of creating a life I didn't want. I decided to stop drinking, convinced that this was the leading cause of all my problems. I couldn't do it independently, so it became a detox clinic. There, they found my problems fundamental and advised me to work on them after completing the detox within a clinical psychotherapeutic department. Relapse was otherwise virtually inevitable. It wasn't an easy decision. My wife wanted me back at work as soon as possible. I felt like an emotional wreck but, at the same time, responsible for my family. Contrary to my expectations, the relationship problems had become worse since I was sober. I couldn't see how it was going to continue. That was probably what ultimately made me decide to continue my treatment. The film *One Flew Over the Cuckoo's Nest* was about the only image I had of a psychiatric admission.

Fortunately, the (new to me) world I ended up in was different. It was the first time in my life that I experienced such a feeling of safety and gentleness towards me. At first, it was mainly a matter of getting used to it. However, as seems to be in my nature, it soon became '*hasta la victoria siempre*'. All problems would and had to be banished from my world once and for all.

I found the group psychotherapy strange. The therapist hardly reacted, and you had to ensure you got your story across. The goal was clear to me; the path to it was anything but. Speaking freely was difficult for me. All my life, I have learned that everything you say can (and will) be used against you. However, the stories of my fellow group members regularly gave me something in return. Creative therapy was much easier for me with drawing, painting, etc. I hardly felt the inner resistance to expose myself, and I quickly came into contact with what, for me, hidden, lived within me. Yet it didn't remain easy. Treasure hunting without a map – that's what it sometimes looked like the most.

While I initially assumed I had to change because of my wife and family, after a few months of admission, I could no longer get around the fact that I would never be able to meet my wife's expectations. The inevitable consequence was divorce. For me, this was a serious low point. That's how a gambler must feel when he has bet everything on one horse and loses. There was nothing left to live for. In hindsight, the care with which I was surrounded by the department and the support the various therapies and therapists gave me at the time was my salvation.

There was no way back, so I continued on my chosen path. I made progress (although it was often barely noticeable to me). I learned to know myself better and better. I discovered, for example, where the roots of my allergy to authoritarian men and my weakness for women in need lay. I also learned that I had and was allowed to have boundaries. I realised I did not expect others to be perfect, so I could not or did not have to be either. It became 'for those who love me, I will be named'. Gradually, it became clear to me that I had flaws and gifts. The old mechanisms had not suddenly disappeared and were often faster and stronger than the newly acquired knowledge. Yet it was not being blind anymore that helped to avoid the same pitfalls over and over again.

After a year-and-a-half of full-time admission through a short tapering-off in day admission, I was back to reality. The psychotherapy was continued through weekly individual sessions with the psychologist who had supervised the group therapy. In the meantime, I had a regular appointment with the psychiatrist in whom I had come to have great confidence.

Things went reasonably well, in contrast to what I had experienced. After a relatively short relationship, I lived alone. I had given up hope and belief in 'love'. Not drinking worked without help. I built a new life from the useable remains of my previous life, with the big difference that this time, it was my life. It felt like liberation.

After a few months, I gradually started working again. My workplace was still there, but the job content had become an empty box. I was on the road for three-and-a-half hours daily, doing hardly anything for eight hours. This was unbearable for me, and there was no hope of improvement. So I looked for and found other work. The new work suited me well. However, my workload gradually grew. I did signal that it was beyond my abilities, but I managed to make everything work every time, and as a result, I was not heard. I thought I was guarding my boundaries but constantly went far beyond them. During this period, I had recurring dreams in which I ended up in a hopeless situation that became more and more hopeless the harder I tried to solve it until there was nothing left but to wake up.

The weekly appointments with the psychologist brought no clarification. There was only the quote that life was a struggle for everyone, but for some, more than others. Again, I had ended up in a life beyond my means and found no help or way out. Disappointed, I stopped the psychotherapy and took a flight forward again. This did not improve things, and it meant a re-admission to the detox clinic.

In the meantime, despite a relatively active social life, I was regularly confronted with moments of loneliness. There were enough people in my life, but I missed someone with whom I could share a piece of my life. The psychiatrist suggested that I sign up on a dating site. I didn't feel like it myself, but I was convinced that he had my best interests at heart, and after lighting a candle in Compostela and Lourdes, I decided to try anyway.

After going through many profiles and a few dates that came to nothing, I contacted someone with whom it could become 'something'. It felt right, but I was afraid that it was too good to be true, that, as in the past, I was taking my dreams for reality. This dichotomy in my head grew as we got to know each other better. Together with the exhaustion as a result of my work, this led to a few short crisis admissions.

Ultimately, I became convinced of the relationship. I had to stop my work out of necessity, which is now called burnout. This resulted in a more extended admission to day therapy. Given my age (I was then fifty), the aim was to get back to work still. I followed specialised trajectory guidance to understand in which direction I could still look for a possible career change (I had tried the most diverse jobs and statuses). I stopped the day of admission on the understanding that the psychotherapy would still be continued. Individual conversations with a psychologist were not financially feasible for me as a single person with a replacement income. It became a discussion group in a mental health care centre.

After a relatively short time (a few months), I had to conclude that this was bringing me very little, and, in consultation with the doctor, I also stopped it. The trajectory guidance had also been completed, and the sentence in the final report, '… he still wants to but can't anymore', said it all for me. It took me some time, but I decided to accept the situation and try to make the best of it.

At this moment, I have a calm but well-filled, satisfying, imperfect life with my wife, who has become the love of my life. Worse and better periods alternate, but the threatening black hole I once struggled with stays away. The real change in how I look at myself and the world around me started during my clinical psychotherapeutic admission. It is clear to me that psychotherapy has yielded a lot, although I have to admit that I have experienced it as a complex and slow process. A process that is never finished. Do I find everything solved with it? Certainly not. However, when I do the exercise and look back on where I came from, I cannot but see that I would never have gotten this far without that help.

Sometimes, I regret not having sought and found help twenty years earlier. As long as no new developments in my life jeopardise the stability I have achieved, I do not need to go any further. I still have a regular appointment with my psychiatrist. Knowing that there is someone I can always turn to gives me a sense of security. Looking to the future, I hope it can stay that way.

14 I.D.

A combination of a stressful work situation and health problems with my youngest son led to my crash seven years ago, but I had been living with too much stress for years. At work, I combined too many tasks and worked more than full-time. Nevertheless, I failed to complete all my assignments on time. I also never dared to refuse the request to do extra work.

My youngest son had been having problems with his stomach and intestines for a few months and was admitted to the hospital for tests. These did not reveal anything, and the doctors suspected that it was a psychosomatic complaint (two years later, a different diagnosis came out). After a conversation with the psychologist, she told us that my son had said that he was sorry that his mum was always so stressed. This broke my heart, and I decided to make an appointment with a psychiatrist. Shortly after that appointment, I collapsed.

On the prescription of my GP, I had been taking an antidepressant for a few years. On the day of my breakdown, he prescribed two weeks' rest. I got an appointment with the psychiatrist and then with a psychodrama therapist. The psychiatrist thought that my biggest problem was a lack of assertiveness and that this would be the most suitable therapy for me. However, during my sick leave, I had already slipped further. I started smoking and hurting myself. When I told the therapist about my condition, she advised me to go to the psychiatric ward (PWGH) for a short admission. I was depressed, had no energy left at all, and felt both mentally and physically completely exhausted. I had sleep problems, was constantly worrying and brooding, could no longer concentrate and was overwhelmed by excessive feelings of guilt, both towards my work and towards my family. I was trembling all over my body and cutting into my fingers.

I was admitted twice in a row for eight weeks to the PWGH. During the second admission, I received electroconvulsive therapy (ECT) but without result. I was referred for admission to a psychotherapeutic centre. As a result of this decision, I started hurting myself even more. This admission lasted five months, after which I followed outpatient therapy again with the psycho-drama therapist. I also went back to work part-time. It was only in this admission that I had brought up the sexual abuse from my childhood with the trainee psychologist, and those memories kept haunting me.

Soon after, I was urgently readmitted to the PWGH. In the meantime, I also had suicidal thoughts. In the PWGH, both the psychologist and the psychiatrist tried to convince me to tell my mother about the sexual abuse by my father. After having had several short admissions again (including after a suicide attempt), I agreed to a referral to a psychiatric hospital (PH). According to the PWGH, they could no longer do anything for me as long as I did not have a conversation with my mother. I felt let down by everyone. During the last admissions, I also began to regularly have panic attacks, with trembling all over my body.

After a week in a short-stay ward, I was immediately transferred to a clin-ical psychotherapeutic ward in the same PH. This was yet another blow for me. With each admission, I had the idea that it would be of short duration and constantly put pressure on myself to return to work as soon as possible and take care of my family. From my first admission to the PWGH, I mini-mised my problems in comparison to those of the other patients. I also had difficulty accepting the illness and blamed myself for being ill. I saw it as a conscious choice and considered myself a weak faker. This certainly hindered the road to recovery.

Even in the PWGH, it became clear that group psychotherapy was not my thing. I am naturally not a big talker, and certainly not in a group. I usually only speak up when asked a question. In the psychotherapeutic centre, the psychologist also involved the people who did not spontaneously take the floor by asking them questions himself. Through these questions, I managed to tell something in the group. I once attended a presentation on resilience and burden (the backpack we all carry) that made me start thinking more about the abuse by my father in my youth. This was sexual abuse, emotional abuse and physical violence. I began to realise that my problems might not be solely due to the stress at work and the health problems of my son. I then mentioned this to the trainee psychologist after she had promised not to tell anyone else. I opened a box that was hard to close again at that moment ...

After this more prolonged admission, I also told the psychodrama thera-pist, the psychiatrist and the psychologist in the PWGH about the abuse. However, little was done with it, primarily because of me. At the PWGH, they said I could only get better if I told my mother, which was not an option for me. I was afraid that I would lose both my mother and father and that my mother would be unhappy for the rest of her life.

In the clinical psychotherapeutic treatment that followed, my childhood problems were worked on extensively. I learned to see the consequences the abuse had on the rest of my life, on my marriage, on who I was and on my problems. Halfway through my admission, I was already referred to a psychoanalytic therapist outside the hospital to have individual psychotherapy there. This has helped me a lot. To this day, I still go there twice a week for a conversation.

Towards the end of my admission, the psychiatrist, the psychologist and the nursing staff convinced me to tell the story of my childhood to my then-husband. He was asking many questions about the numerous and/or lengthy treatments. After much hesitation, I told him. I still wonder if this was a good decision. Six months later, he admitted that he no longer liked me and that he wanted to divorce … Later, he said that he had been struggling with his feelings for a year (since the beginning of my admission to the PH) but that he had not dared to say anything because he feared that I would have a relapse again.

During my admissions, I have significantly benefited from trainee psychologists. In the psychotherapeutic centre, there was only contact with the psychologist during the group therapies. With the trainee psychologist, on the other hand, there was weekly individual contact, and I was able to have good conversations. This is also how I could confide my 'secret' from my childhood to her. It was probably not a good idea to make her promise not to tell anyone else on the staff …

I didn't click with the psychologist in the later clinical psychotherapeutic ward. He often said barely a word, and ensuring you got your story across was up to you. The goal had to come from yourself, something I'm not good at. With the trainee psychologist, I did manage to have good conversations and speak openly and freely. Was this due to her different approach, because she was a woman, or because the conversations with her were more frequent? Probably a combination of these factors. Unfortunately, her internship ended after about three months. She was also present during the group therapy.

During the final group therapy session in her presence, I shared the story of my childhood. Until then, no one in my group had been aware of it. I wanted to tell my story while she was still there, so that she could support me if necessary. After that group session, the staff assumed I would continue to speak up in the group therapies, but without the presence of the trainee psychologist, I couldn't manage it anymore.

After around four months of inpatient treatment, the psychiatrist advised me to start therapy with an external psychologist. My first question to her was whether she used the same approach as the hospital psychologist. It soon became clear, thankfully, that this was not the case. It took some time, but our conversations gradually became meaningful, and I grew to trust her completely. By asking targeted questions without putting me under pressure, she helped me talk about everything. When I tried to recall memories of my childhood and my father, I kept hitting a figurative wall – I couldn't say anything and would suffer panic attacks. But she always managed to calm me down, and at a certain point, I was finally able to talk about the sexual abuse.

It was mainly the one-on-one conversations with the trainee psychologist, the nursing staff, the psychiatrist, the social worker, and the external psychologist that helped me make progress. I've always been sporty, but for a long time I was no longer able to exercise. The physical activities in the psychiatric hospital did me good, though they also confronted me with how poor my condition had become. In the 'trauma' group – a small group – I did manage to tell my story, unlike in the larger group therapies. The small setting and the sense that others had experienced something similar probably made it easier.

Listening to music during music therapy also felt good, and the songs gave me a way to express myself in the group. Making music or singing, however, made me shut down. Listening to music on my smartphone brought me a lot of comfort throughout all my admissions. I had a fixed playlist – my 'musical pharmacy'. Occupational therapy wasn't really my thing, but I did a lot of colouring, which helped calm my mind. As I'm not at all assertive, I attended several assertiveness training sessions. I found the theory very interesting, but I wasn't able to carry out the practical exercises or role plays.

A close contact or friendship with someone in my group who had also been a victim of sexual abuse certainly helped me as well. We didn't always have in-depth conversations about the abuse, but because we shared the same issue, we connected. We were able to laugh together and grieve together as well.

After this most recent admission, I gradually returned to work. After a difficult period, there came a moment when I once again felt my employer's trust in me. That helped a great deal in regaining some self-confidence and a sense of purpose. In total, I was in clinical psychotherapy for eight months: the first half full-time, the second half in day therapy. During and after day therapy, I continued to see the external psychologist twice a week – and I still do. I tried reducing it to once a week, but I found that only everyday issues were discussed, and there was no longer any real depth. I also still attend monthly sessions with the psychiatrist for process support.

My divorce most likely delayed my treatment and made the recovery process more difficult. For a long time, grief overshadowed everything. After each longer admission, I felt as though I were 'cured'. But through trial and error, I've come to understand that ongoing outpatient treatment is essential.

Throughout psychotherapy, I've gained insight into who I am and what my strengths and weaknesses are. I've also come to realise how much the consequences of the abuse have affected the rest of my life. I can now speak with both the psychologist and the psychiatrist about my difficult childhood and its effects without trembling, shaking, or crying (although the tears are still never far away). I've also learned that it was no small thing to carry 'the secret' on my own for so long – it had a significant mental and physical impact on me. I've come to realise that my marriage wasn't all sunshine and roses. We mainly had problems when it came to sex. For me, sex always felt like a duty

– something I only did to meet the needs of my ex-husband. During sex, I would always see images of my naked father, which caused me to freeze.

It took a while, but I believe I've now been free of depressive symptoms for about six months. The wish to die, the suicidal thoughts, and the urge to self-harm lingered for a long time, but they are truly a thing of the past. During my admissions and especially after my divorce, I gained a lot of weight. Two years ago, I started exercising again and made changes to my eating habits. I've now lost over twenty kilograms. Exercising and losing weight have given me a better self-image. I feel that I've regained greater resilience and more self-confidence. I feel pretty well these days.

Even so, I still need the sessions with the psychologist. I want to reduce them to once a week later this year, as it remains quite an expense. I've slowly started working more and would like to return to full-time employment. I still struggle with feelings of guilt towards my children. I feel that I abandoned them for a time due to my lengthy hospital admissions. The fear of a new depression, along with the urge to self-harm and suicidal thoughts, is still present. There are still many unanswered questions.

During my clinical psychotherapeutic admission, I once saw a sex scene involving two women on television, which aroused me. After my divorce, I did some experimenting and once paid a woman for sex. That felt wonderful to me. Later, I also paid a man for sex. I wasn't aroused, and it felt like a chore. I continued to see the woman regularly, and it felt better than anything I'd ever experienced with a man. However, due to the COVID-19 pandemic, it has now been months since we last met. I don't miss it and don't feel the need for sexual arousal. At the moment, I don't know whether I'll see her again.

I think that in future, therapy will need to focus mainly on relational aspects, alongside the daily worries and concerns (work, children, housing, etc.) that cause me stress. I'll also need to remain aware of my pitfalls, such as a lack of assertiveness and the tendency to want to please everyone. I'll have to keep listening to my body, so I can take action when tension builds and it all becomes too much.

15 J.D.

I was eighteen and struggling with anorexia. I knew it had to stop. My body was suffering too much. After about a year, I managed to stop it. Without any help, without talking to anyone about it. I always thought I was in control of my life. That I was steering the course. I felt the pressure to perform well. I wanted to be a good daughter, a good friend, a good partner, a good mother, a good employee. Always 100 per cent committed, cheerful and ready to help others. By carefully planning my path, I thought I would avoid setbacks. I found a good partner, we had two children, and I'd worked for the same employer in a management position for eighteen years. Everything seemed to be going well until I completely blocked. I was thirty-nine and overwhelmed, paralysed by fear.

I always thought: depression, that won't happen to me! I persevere, I am a fighter, I don't give up. Until it happens to you. For days and weeks, fighting against my feelings. I don't want this! You can hold on for a while, but not for long. All senses are on high alert ... light, sound, taste, all come in so intensely. Overwhelmed, exhausted! I was admitted to the city PWGH ward. This was followed by six months of outpatient therapy. I recovered pretty quickly. I stopped working at my job and started working elsewhere progressively. I completely weaned myself off my medication with the psychiatrist and didn't make a new appointment. I didn't click with my psychologist, so I stopped seeing them entirely, too. Proud as punch. I've done it! I'm over it!

Until I got stuck again after six months, I struggled with my emotions again and was overwhelmed by fear. I completely seized up physically. My body cramped several times. I couldn't think logically anymore. I didn't even know how to drive a car anymore. My body set off all the alarm bells inside me. No matter how hard I fought my second depression, it didn't go away; it just got worse. At that point, you're very searching and vulnerable. Finding the right people and not some 'coach' (without proper training) is essential. In times of depression and anxiety, only a good psychiatrist, psychologist and the right setting can provide relief. This is a crucial phase in the treatment, where you realise that a thorough approach is needed. I am, therefore, very grateful that I put myself on the waiting list for the PH during that phase. After a waiting period, I was admitted to the clinic. You do not know what will happen with your suitcase in the car park.

I started with full inpatient admission. No joke! A room of my own? Not possible for now. A room with two ... unpleasant, cold, strange smell. Everything you don't want. I found it very difficult, but you want to be helped, so you adapt. Even though you're an inpatient, you go home on Wednesdays and weekends. Very important. I'm lucky to have a warm family and good friends who supported me 100 per cent. Crucial, in my opinion, during this challenging process. An important and, for me, difficult phase was accepting the depression. I learned not to fight it but to give it a place. To try to understand where it came from.

The clinic is a place where they work hard to find out how you can best express yourself. Musical expression, body expression, visual expression and verbal therapy are just a few options. I'm verbally strong, so I benefited most from the sessions with the psychologist and psychiatrist. Gradually, your own story comes to the surface.

I have to admit that the group sessions were often hard for me. I wanted to find more like-minded people with a similar story to mine. This wasn't the case. I quickly learned that everyone's story is unique. Sometimes, it was difficult to hear the stories of fellow patients. I felt I had to help them or encourage them. At first, I also didn't understand why the psychologist didn't participate more actively during psychotherapy. Now I realise that this is deliberate, that everyone's story is allowed to 'be'. Articulating this story without anyone judging or interfering builds trust and makes everything discussable. They listen without judging.

I often found the sessions where you get theoretical explanations about psychotherapy enlightening. You get explanations about parentification, mentalisation, different disorders, and cause and effect. It is necessary to trace your own story. One session applies to yourself; the other doesn't.

You're also asked to write your life story. Writing brought me much clarity; it's a form of processing. The beauty of psychotherapy is that you get the time to come to your insights. Only then can you fully grasp them. At the beginning of the therapy, I could get annoyed by the 'passive' attitude of the psychotherapist. I thought, 'I'm here now – just help me – just tell me what I have to do'. I was incredibly clinging and wanted answers. Now I realise I had to come to the necessary insights and that this is the only right way. Psychotherapy is mainly something you have to do yourself. The psychiatrist, psychologist and the whole team are there for you and set you on your way, but you must do the hard work yourself.

Those who are willing to work, to toil, to fail and to start again will succeed. A very friendly professional team is there to support you and provide a safe framework.

Because psychotherapy demands a lot from you, there are also relaxing elective sessions. These included philosophy, body and mind in balance, dance, relaxation, mindfulness and intuitive painting. Philosophy did me good. Often, therapy is such a close zoom-in of yourself that it does you good to zoom out and search for the bigger picture of life.

You could often find me in my free time in the art studio with G. Escaping into art and escaping the heaviness the clinic brings. Discovering the childlike freedom within yourself. Unlike the occupational therapy sessions, where I felt patronised, the studio was a place of creation. G. is not a therapist but an artist who gives you much freedom. Her humour and laughter will stay with me. This was my outlet during this challenging period. My escape route.

I stayed there for six months in full inpatient admission. After that, I followed weeks of day therapy at the clinic. Then you're at home and go to the clinic on weekdays from nine to five.

When I entered the PH, I thought I would stay for a maximum of one month. It's human to want to put a time limit on it, preferably a very short one. It quickly became apparent that this would take much longer. I could move forward only when I let go of the 'timing'.

Describing what happened during that period in the clinic is very difficult. It's something you undergo. You can't 100 per cent explain what you're doing there. It happens to you. Your bewilderment is given space. You're drawn into the programme, which is hugely demanding. It even takes over your life for a while. Frightening.

It's essential to stop at the clinic on time. You mustn't get stuck in it. It takes much courage to step in but just as much courage to step out. At a certain point, you have to detach yourself from this very caring framework and apply the insights you've learned to your daily life. Psychotherapy is gaining insight into yourself and the patterns you're stuck in. After the insight comes the changing of those patterns. As my psychiatrist always put it beautifully: 'It's as if, after years of driving a car in the same way, they suddenly tell you that you have to do it completely differently.' Indeed, it is not easy, but it is necessary. Only upon leaving do the puzzle pieces become a little more explicit.

After the full inpatient admission and day therapy, my outpatient therapy followed. The clinic recommended a good psychologist to me. It's so important that there is further follow-up when you close the clinic door. Attending a psychologist is not financially feasible for everyone, which is a pity. Those sessions are critical to me. The story doesn't end at the clinic; it only begins. Weekly, completely open, saying what's bothering you, what makes you feel good, what makes you grow, expressing emotions, articulating fears, continuing to grow in therapy and, above all, continuing to grow as a person and knowing that someone is listening without judging. Do you feel that you are no longer alone? This outpatient therapy is still ongoing, and I don't plan to stop it.

In short, I can say that clinical psychotherapy helped me to put together and understand my own story. I learned that my own positive and negative emotions are allowed to have a place in my life and that I don't have to fight them. I learned to say 'no' and to express my anger. I knew that parentification applies to me. In my childhood, I reacted sensitively to the emotional needs of my parents. This happened very unconsciously and spontaneously. My own needs and feelings faded into the background. Over the years, these piled up. They manifested in my anorexia, but I didn't realise that at the time. My two depressions were also at the root of years of ignoring my feelings. The moment I allowed my feelings in, it felt like a tsunami washing over me. My stay in the PH became a real struggle. I learned that I think and process the emotions of others too much for them – something I shouldn't do. Throughout my admission, my balance was completely disrupted. Once the process has started, you can't go back. It's also complicated to explain what you're going through to your relatives and how much it demands of you. You must be given the time to go through this process. It's also vital that the environment (my family) is involved in your process. For example, I remember the consultation with the psychiatrist and my husband. During admission, you often become even more profound than you were before. My husband was distraught during that phase. Then you need a psychiatrist who stays calm and explains to the environment, but also to yourself and points out that this is a normal phase in the recovery process. The children could join some sessions where they received explanations at their level about 'where is your mummy now', 'what is a psychiatrist', etc. They also got a tour of the building. I'm very grateful that time was also made for them. By involving children and partners, they can better frame the whole event. It's difficult for the patient and profoundly impactful for the entire family.

Medication is another point. Before my admission, I was against medication. I found it difficult to accept that I had to take it. In the meantime, I've revised my opinion on this. Medication was essential for me. However, I want to add that, in my opinion, this can only be prescribed by a good psychiatrist, and follow-up is necessary.

It's now four years since my discharge from the PH. I still go to my psychiatrist and psychologist every two months. I feel good. Normal. I'm so grateful for what psychotherapy has given me. I have so much more insight into myself, understand and see specific patterns and am proud that I have broken certain patterns. I no longer live in my own shadow but live to the full. Better and wiser because of psychotherapy … I can actually (although cautiously) answer 'yes' to that.

16 J.D.C.

I wasn't a good student at secondary school; I was a bit of a free spirit who loved building dens in nature and spending most of my time tinkering in my grandfather's workshop. I was primarily a hands-on person, curious about the meaning of life. I also wondered why I study. What's the point? I was a searcher, internally conflicted without realising it. Concentrating and sitting still at a desk weren't options. My parents were at their wits' end with me. Many conflicts with teachers formed the undercurrent. I also attended many construction camps in the Eastern Bloc, where I learned about bricklaying, concrete-making and building churches.

At eighteen, my body had already shown signs of fatigue. The GP couldn't immediately explain it. I was admitted to a general hospital for two weeks – no follow-up or diagnosis, except a suggestion to see a psychologist. I never followed up on this out of shame, ignorance and denial. My aunt (whom I could confide in) noticed something was wrong but couldn't delve deeper. So she suggested I go to a 'counsellor'. Eventually, I ended up with a hypnotist. After a few sessions, I stopped. Through my aunt, I later joined a Tarot working group. I got many questions but few answers. Many unusual people tried to manipulate my energy but, as quacks, they did me more harm than good.

I wandered the streets, restless, nervous and constantly busy setting up various projects. I didn't know what I wanted. I had my mopeds and the cellar where I retreated. School friends, who had a bad influence on me, came along. They taught me to smoke, drink and do many things that shouldn't see the light of day. I rebelled against authority at school and in the scouts and regularly clashed with teachers. The school counsellors tried to help, but it remained unclear why I exhibited such defiant behaviour. I was suspended for 'negative leadership' in the scouts for a year. I had become unmanageable, an *enfant terrible*. I was full of sorrow and a deep longing for the time I grew up as a child with my grandparents. Unbeknownst to me, I suffered enormously from a longing for my idealised childhood years. I missed something precious or essential that was there before: lots of attention, endless love and excessive admiration from my grandparents. In retrospect, I was processing a significant loss. This started when my grandmother died when I was twelve and intensified at sixteen after the death of my beloved grandfather. Because of this, I was deeply saddened, gloomy, unhappy and misunderstood. I sought attention in the wrong way and thus exhausted myself.

When I came of age and was no longer subject to compulsory schooling, I developed an inferiority complex because I hadn't studied enough. I felt I was missing something ... I decided to attend weekend school for electronics. I combined this with a daytime industrial sciences course, preparing for engineering studies. I was at my desk seven days a week. I was motivated and intensely interested in mathematics, physics and chemistry. When I graduated, I got back in touch with an old scout leader who lived in Canada. He invited me for a two-month holiday on his old farm. Before leaving for Canada, I went on a construction camp in Ukraine. I left for Canada without having caught my breath. I did long cycling trips alone, with little luggage and shelter. I slept under trees, on the beach and at people's homes. The journey was long and exhausting, braving much wind and rain. I returned from Canada and started my engineering studies. I was nervous, suffered from a fear of failure and found it difficult to sleep. Fatigue set in; I was utterly exhausted. I had pushed my body and mind to the limit. Without realising it, I started having my first hallucinations. Concentrating became impossible, and I couldn't even draw a simple line on paper. At that time, I was looking to become independent from home. I had a strong desire to become self-sufficient. I lived above the garage at my aunt's house during that period. Her daughter was then doing her first year of internship in psychiatry. She interviewed me and listened to my complaints. Inexperienced and thoughtless, she went to the pharmacy with me. We came out with a bottle of Haldol drops. I would have the dose in my own hands and use it myself. I was ignorant and saw no dangers. I stopped going to classes, became restless and started wandering around. I suddenly got the idea to look up my first girlfriend. I heard she had moved into her place. She was furnishing and renovating her little house. I was refused entry by her sister, who said she didn't want to see me. I got angry and threw stones at the windows and doors. I was losing myself. That day, I took many more Haldol drops because of the crisis. I stumbled through the streets and started seeing horrible scenes in my head. A severe psychosis had occurred, and my mother had to rush me to the hospital. There, I caused chaos in the emergency room. I didn't know what was happening to me. Medication was administered, and a little later, I woke up in the Emergency Psychiatric Centre. I couldn't understand what had happened to me. After two weeks, I was transferred to a more specialised hospital where psychotherapy was the main focus. The beginning of a long recovery process had begun without me knowing or wanting it at the time. I thought I would be recovered after a couple of months, but they couldn't give a clear timeframe. I had taken on too much, but how had it come to this? I couldn't understand that talking and digging deeper would solve my problem. There was no alternative but to cooperate and do what was expected of me. I had never chosen to go to a therapist just like that. What do you think: 'I'm not crazy!'

When I first met my psychotherapist, and he started calmly asking interesting questions, I immediately felt at ease. Finally, someone with whom I could freely share and tell everything was something new for me. He reminded me more of a good friend or my grandfather. Somehow, trust was established, which was necessary for the process. There was a mystique about him; he seemed progressive in his vision and approach. I liked that; he had a plan, I thought. He could also surprisingly act like a good father figure with sound advice, for example, when I was in a marital crisis many years later. He also encouraged me to continue my engineering studies and attend an academy. We achieved good results step by step, so the therapy integrated itself into my life as a fixed value.

Curiously, I began to attach myself and develop a valuable bond. This made it more difficult to distance myself from a kind of 'guru' in my mind. Therefore, autonomous thinking and detaching from the therapist often came up. At first, he is a stranger, gradually a companion on the journey. Whether he walks in front of, beside or behind you is never clear, but he is always there with full attention.

I experienced psychotherapy as a kind of 'sacred space'. Nowhere had I delved deeply into the essence and my many unresolved questions. Free association and thinking aloud were initially helpful to get things going. Putting my emotions into words was initially tricky, but I learned to do that. There was progressive insight, constantly building on a foundation that had now been firmly laid. Such a solid building block doesn't come quickly; you must undergo a period of resistance – of searching, digging, not understanding and talking it through. Once you've talked about a particular topic enough and looked at it from all angles, that piece becomes part of yourself again.

Previously unknown and suppressed, a stone comes back to the surface. You then use it to place your foot, searching for the next loose foundation. At a certain point, 'almost' everything is clear, and you know yourself. From then on, you can almost predict and observe how you will react to a particular situation and why exactly that emotion will occur. But how do you deal with the combination of self-knowledge and less positive emotions? The powerlessness is the most challenging part because you want to change it, but you can't just do it. After a while, you realise that changing isn't possible, but you accept it.

There is a specific order in the whole process. You first seek wisdom, insight and knowledge. Psychotherapy can be beneficial for this. You then use that knowledge to distinguish between what you can and cannot change. You try to accept the things you cannot change. That doesn't happen overnight. You need the 'courage' to do what you can change. That's the mindset to stop an old pattern.

What helped a lot was the insight and process of becoming independent. I want to detach myself from home, specifically from my mother. I moved out, started working, learned to cook and care for myself. I also worked with certain symbols and metaphors in my sculpture training. Specific problems were sometimes too abstract for me, so I needed to give them plastic form in the specific accompanying material. Being creatively involved with art certainly helped me in my search for depth. In art, I also learned that the result should not be a goal but a journey towards it. Art can and should remain a quest. Similarly, it is reassuring that the psychotherapeutic process will never be finished. It was never dull or monotonous. Certain concepts, emotions, knots, crossties and stumbling blocks were discussed repeatedly. It is a kind of 'mantra sequence' with numerous variations and perspectives.

Given many words and thoughts, insight usually only comes after a session. These insights often come unexpectedly, like a thief in the night. Sometimes, I regret not having written them down or kept them somewhere. These insights are deep inside you but partly covered with a sheet. They can become very clear during a conversation, and you don't have time to write them down in your report. You go outside, and all the insights are suddenly gone. I would like to reread my insights and searches and reflect on my reference work. At school, I was never good at attending class and paying attention to the board. I always had to write down my study material in different forms, using diagrams and drawings to summarise insights. In this way, the insights obtained from the theory became a part of myself. I would have liked to have written the summaries during the process as a point of reference and result. A personal database that you can always access via an app when you lose your way seems helpful to me and would give me more peace of mind.

My first session started when I was twenty-three and led to a full-time admission of one year. This was followed by a year of day therapy. As I continued to build my life afterwards, I attended weekly outpatient group therapy. After a while, it became individual sessions in private practice. Those moments gave me structure, security and a foothold. I am writing this testimony at the age of fifty-three, as I am nearing completion. But stopping is also tricky because you must end a long-standing, trusting relationship. There were intermittent breaks. There were also periods of more frequent consultations during difficult times. There was always a tailored schedule according to needs. Custom-made!

The process took about thirty years because I ask many questions. I am also highly driven to learn and very curious by nature. Many challenges have arisen, in which I have found much strength in the constant psychotherapeutic approach and insights. My personality may be too complex. Insights took a long time to sink in properly. You don't easily break a good trusting relationship because it provides comfort in your head. Psychotherapy or long-term thinking wasn't even a choice but, for me, an absolute necessity.

Much has changed, and at the same time, nothing. By that, I mean I have remained who I am, but the sharp edges have been smoothed off. Deep down, I stay the same person with my characteristics. Good and less good character traits are better known. What is different is that I know much better how to deal with the emotions that arise around the core problem because they are very recognisable in daily life. In a conflict, I will be quicker to concede when the problem lies with me. Even if the problem doesn't lie with me, this will be clearer quickly. This also allows me to engage in dialogue more calmly and constructively. Now that I have explored all my rooms, holes and crevices to the deepest corners, it gives me a rock-solid foundation. Above all, it gives me peace of mind, serenity, and clarity. This was the 'essence' of psychotherapy for me. Before, there was much fog, unrest, fear, uncertainty, anger, exhaustion …

In terms of problems, there was a massive difference between the upbringing of my grandparents and that of my parents. On the one hand, I enjoyed the admiration of my grandparents. I received a lot of attention and love there. Everything I created was beautiful! I was their god. I had my little world there, and nobody was allowed to disturb it. In my fantasy, I protected my built paradise by building a colossal castle around it. In contrast, my father was somewhat absent and paid less attention to me. He came up with rules and punishments at every opportunity. He didn't understand me or know what was happening inside me. My mother continued to treat me like a child, even at a later age, so that I couldn't grow up as a man. My older sister was very dominant and belittling. This created in me a craving for attention and admiration. This caused numerous peculiar phenomena and counterreactions to normal functioning. Result: exhaustion, anger, envy, quickly transitioning to an irritated emotional state if something appears to stand in the way of that admiration. Always looking for a haven and wanting to protect it at all costs.

Psychotherapy is like speleology for me. The speleologist is the guide-therapist who will explore all the nooks and crannies of the cave together with and through the patient. The cave is full of mirrors in unexpected, unnoticed and astonishing places. The cave is a branching network of countless passages, crevices and cavities. Extended like the roots of a tree. The chambers are the places of events from your past. They are repressed, hidden and lie under a thick layer of sand or dust. All these caverns are exposed during the process, resembling a significant cleaning spread over a long period. Don't forget that speleology is a risky activity. It would be irresponsible to venture into it without equipment or an experienced person. The therapist is experienced and ensures that you never get stuck or trapped. He knows the cave, which parts can flood, and where the loose fragments are. He lets the patient walk around and asks questions about the why and how of their search. Why take a particular path, and especially why not take a specific path? The most common danger in speleology is falling. Uncontrolled jumping and sliding down slopes must be avoided to reduce the risk of falling.

Therefore, the step-by-step slow psychotherapeutic process is fundamental. It is safe to put your feet back on a previously unsteady stone but, by talking about it, you have restabilised it with the right 'cement'.

17 K.D.V.

I started therapy because I felt stuck in my life. My father's death (suicide) had a profound impact on me. I was thirteen at the time, and I felt incredibly sad and helpless. I couldn't talk to anyone about it. My grief led to regular feelings of guilt and shame. It was the most intense emotion I've ever experienced. My depression was melancholic. Further life problems included sexual abuse at the age of twenty. After the birth of my daughter, I suffered from postnatal depression, coupled with a difficult marriage with an authoritarian partner, causing me to withdraw increasingly. Eventually, I attempted suicide several times.

My first contact with psychiatric help was a referral from my GP to a psychiatrist at a general hospital. At one point, I was too melancholic to continue as an outpatient, and admission became necessary on her advice. When you're entirely non-functional and a danger to yourself (severe suicidal thoughts), staying at home is no longer an option. Because I was so ill, I didn't realise this myself. I didn't want to be admitted because I didn't know what it entailed. It was drastic, but there was no other way.

At that time, I had severe sleep problems: insomnia and no more day-night rhythm. Or reversing day and night. Low energy. Suicidal thoughts. Worrying. Cognitive problems: concentration problems/indecisiveness. I thought I was losing my mind. I no longer enjoyed things I used to love. I also had little interaction with family and friends and no longer desired social contact. I isolated myself, staying home as much as possible and neglecting myself and my household. I had very low self-esteem: I could no longer function daily.

Honestly, I didn't have high expectations at the start. The world of psychiatry was utterly foreign to me. I had a negative view of it due to negative media coverage. Fortunately, this has improved significantly in recent years thanks to campaigns like 'Too Mad!?' (Dutch: *Te Gek*), the 10-Day Mental Health campaign, and Red Nose Day for young people. I thought psychiatry was for 'abnormal people', for 'crazy people'. Because of this, I was ashamed to be in psychiatry. It was the world turned upside down: I was seeking treatment for problems I was ashamed of. Furthermore, I felt shame because I was seeking help. Few people knew where I was staying.

At first, psychotherapy was very difficult for me. Because of my attitude (very closed off, distant) and my mindset (little hope for improvement and, therefore, little talking), my psychotherapy was very slow. The start of my psychiatric treatment was also the start of my introduction to psychotherapy. Group therapy, in particular, was extra unpleasant for me, as was the process guidance with the psychiatrist: I come from a family where there was no culture of talking about problems, let alone about taboo subjects like my father's suicide and sexuality. I didn't receive sex education at school; I never received any … When you've lived in that 'culture of silence' for years, you don't suddenly start pouring everything out in a group.

Initially, building a good relationship with my psychiatrist was challenging; I was very closed off. I was also a little afraid of him because he could put me under strict supervision, preventing me from leaving the centre and subjecting me to much monitoring. I didn't understand that this was for my good; I felt it more like a punishment. After a few consultations, things went more smoothly: I thought he had my best interests at heart and would do everything to improve me. I also initially had a complicated relationship with the psychologist. Challenging group sessions: I didn't dare talk about my problems in a group. It was difficult when someone else talked about their difficulties: sometimes relatable, often weighty stories. I felt I couldn't take it: that my backpack was already full enough. I found it easier to open up to the psychiatric nurse. The distance felt smaller.

Many things helped me during my admission. I'm convinced of that. For example, I attended engaging forum sessions on grief. During my treatment, my bipolar disorder came to light: now that I know I can cope with it much better. Creative and expressive therapy helped the most: it was easier to speak through my creative work. Painting, drawing, making collages … that's my thing. Writing too: writing down my problems is easier than talking about them.

When I was discharged and opted for outpatient treatment (because this was possible at that time), I was followed up for a while by the mobile team: a psychiatric nurse who came to my home every two weeks initially, then once a month. I could discuss with her what was going well and what wasn't. I'm very positive about such initiatives! The connection with the psychiatric hospital wasn't wholly severed: someone was there to follow up and see if I would manage at home. It's interesting to see how such initiatives are evolving and growing. Related to this: aftercare. It's a discussion group of former patients who meet on the last Wednesday evening of each month. A psychiatric nurse facilitates the sessions. I still participate.

The individual sessions with the psychiatrist and psychologist certainly helped, too. Through their years of experience, they quickly gained insight into me as a patient: I sometimes didn't have to say much, yet many of my problems came to the surface, and connections were made that I hadn't realised myself.

During my first admission to a different psychiatric hospital, I was immediately placed in isolation because of suicidal tendencies (including running away). This was a traumatic experience for me. I don't feel that it helped. It made me feel even worse than I already was, and it made me very anxious. I felt like a criminal because it resembled a prison cell. I know that there's a trend within psychiatry to use isolation less. That's a positive development. In the clinical psychotherapeutic ward, I was never placed in an isolation cell; however, I was under increased supervision, which was also not pleasant but necessary at the time.

My psychotherapeutic process lasted about five years – four years of clinical psychotherapy and then another year of psychosocial rehabilitation. The process took much longer than I ever thought it would. The main reason is that I didn't actively participate at the beginning (for the reasons listed above, e.g., not daring to speak in a group). Because of this, I lost much time. Because I was so passive, I remained stagnant for a long time, which is a shame. But I only realised that afterwards.

I went through all the phases: full admission (when it was necessary due to my poor mental state), then day therapy (commuting daily by bus), and, finally, outpatient treatment. Switching to day therapy as soon as possible is advisable: family ties can be rekindled, and it's also good preparation for later discharge. The period of full admission was brutal and should not be under-estimated. I found the admission very intense. It was personally challenging for me to be separated from my family.

I now have more self-confidence and a more positive outlook on life. I dare to be around people again. I now have a favourable view of psychotherapy. I'm much more balanced. I'm wary of mood swings: I can assess myself better in that respect. I have much more self-awareness, making it easier not to fall into the same traps: I have a gentle nature and let people walk all over me too often. Now, I dare to stand up for myself much more. I climbed out of the deep valley and developed my qualities better. I can also be a mother to my daughter (now seventeen) again; we do fun things together. I missed her ter-ribly during my admission – she was much younger then. I felt she was being taken away from me. That was very painful. Besides my illness, I also felt like I had failed as a mother. I can also cope with overstimulation more easily.

Psychotherapy has taught me so much that it's difficult to put into words – self-knowledge and insight into myself. I'm stronger in life. At the beginning, people sometimes say: 'You need to work on yourself.' But what does 'working on yourself' mean? Now I know what it means. The order has brought chaos to my head. During my admission, I lived according to a fixed therapy schedule: this helped bring structure back into my life. The clinic and the psychiatrist saved my life. I've made a very positive evolution. That's for sure. I never would have dared to dream beforehand that I would improve so much through psy-chotherapy. I would recommend psychotherapy to people I meet with mental health problems (people I meet in daily life)! If I ever feel bad again, I will seek help much sooner! Now I know the way to help. I know it exists!

Because I feel better, I look to the future with hope. I don't dare look too far ahead. I've been through too much for that. What makes me feel good is a bal-ance between work and leisure. I work as a volunteer in childcare. I would like to have paid work again. But I have a great fear of whether I will be able to cope. Because of my illness, my relationship ended in divorce. I'm currently single, and I feel good about that. I don't want to burden anyone with my mental health problems. We'll see how it evolves further. I feel much better after my therapy, and I think I can still grow further. Successful experiences can help me with that.

18 K.M.

I was born a very sensitive child, and this has been a recurring theme throughout my life. My parents separated and reunited three times before I turned eight. The first time was for three months, the second for a year, and the third time was final. Each time, I moved with my mother. Every separa-tion was traumatic for me. Three times, I 'lost' my dad, and perhaps 'thanks to' my mother's excellent care, I formed a powerful bond with her at a young age. I 'lost' my dad, and if I lose my mum now, my world will fall apart. This is a reasonably realistic thought, as at that age, an orphan sometimes ends up in a heartless institution without genuine love. My dad only had visiting rights every other Sunday, so he was largely absent throughout my childhood. Even then, I worried about the potential loss of my parents (read: mother), something a child shouldn't have to think about.

During my teens, I was the man of the house. Everything was discussed together, but my mother was strict and always had the final say. Saturday nights were spent at home in front of the television. When I was seventeen, she met my stepfather, whom she eventually married. I was ousted from my position, but I didn't have a problem with that because my stepfather finally let me go out. A new world opened, but I had to be home by one o'clock. I was seventeen and had never been 'out' before. Unfortunately, things didn't work out with him, and after some time, I was kicked out of the house and had to move in with my father. I had three hours to pack everything ...

For a while, I had complete freedom. My father allowed me to do a lot, and suddenly it went from 'home by one' to 'unlimited'. Often arriving home in the morning ... without drugs or anything like that, just having fun! I quickly met a nice girl and was with her for quite some time. But she dreamed of a family and ... staying home in front of the television ... When I started to enjoy my freedom, I would be confined to the house again ... I wasn't ready for a serious relationship, and it ended badly. It was my fault. It was a very painful break-up after two years of ups and downs. That year, my grandfather (my mother's father), with whom I had a good relationship, died, and my mother – on top of the grief of her deceased father – found herself in her second divorce. Her great love. She fell into a very severe depression with often dark thoughts. Suddenly, the care for my mother came to the forefront again. It was a terrible year.

At the end of that year, I attended a concert and was at the front. That was the first time I felt unwell. Oh, a fainting spell or something ... but it repeated itself quickly and more frequently. I developed anxieties and very severe depressive feelings, where I could barely control myself. It was superhuman ... indescribable ... Hell! That's when the long list of doctors, specialists, homoeopathy, hypnosis and so on began ... Nothing helped ... But being admitted to a psychiatric ward is not a tiny step.

My GP initially gave me sick leave with supportive medication. I had to drag myself through the day and, after a month, I was back. I was referred to a neurologist. I remember being given a sample of medication to take in the evening ... Terrible! I slept for fourteen hours straight, and the following day I could barely stand up, completely out of it. I didn't even dare drive my car anymore, and my mother took me back to the doctor. 'There must be something wrong with your nervous system because if I were to take that medication, I wouldn't feel anything,' said the doctor. That treatment was stopped, and then I tried homoeopathy – hours of walking, breathing in the fresh air, and healthy living with supportive homoeopathic medication. I've never spent as much time by the sea as I did then, but the anxiety would return in the evening. I was even afraid to be home alone ... Then, I got the address of a qualified hypnotherapist in Brussels. Yes, I drove to Brussels several times but was never hypnotised – first, introductory conversations and strange questions. The third time, I was supposed to be hypnotised to delve into the past and discover where these anxieties came from. Unfortunately, my condition deteriorated so badly, and in a slight panic, I called the man to ask if it couldn't be sooner. His answer was a huge disappointment. If taking this Tranxene (or something like that) isn't possible, then it will get better ... But it worsened, and something had to be done!

The dark thoughts relentlessly pushed their way through, and it was high time for admission. I never attempted suicide, but I've been close many times. When I arrived, I vividly remember a leaflet stating that anxieties and depression were treated. That gave me a good feeling, and I was completely confident they could help me here. Irrational fears are incomprehensible to many people. Lying in your bed and feeling like your whole room is on fire is inexplicable. I went to a festival with more than sixty thousand people in the summer, and by the end of the same year, I no longer dared to go to an empty café in my street! I expected to be freed from all those terrible symptoms and become the cheerful guy I used to be.

I didn't know about psychoanalysis and didn't believe in it at all. As if 'talking' about your problems would cure you? And of the additional therapies, some were absolutely nothing for me. Cooking, sports, expressive therapy, creative workshop ... I can't remember the exact names anymore, but they're classics. Occupational therapy particularly appealed to me. I'm pretty handy, and I made cupboards, CD racks, and racks for (back then) videotapes and books. Expressive therapy was a disaster, but a pretty, blonde therapist made me skip through the therapy. Creative therapy was a growth process. At first, I never went, but gradually, it appealed to me. I drew the faces of my favourite band (KISS), and the compliments were flattering. It eventually became a favourite pastime.

So, I didn't believe in psychotherapy at all. I started with a negative image but was motivated to become the 'old K.' as quickly as possible. I had to get better. And if talking would help me, then I would do it. When I heard in psychotherapy what other people had experienced, I had the impression that it was much more straightforward for them than for me. For example, rape is a very severe blow to the process. I hadn't experienced any of that. I had the impression that I had a pretty good childhood. But those symptoms of feeling unwell and severe depression were (in themselves) the biggest problem for me. I expected to be cured after a month's admission. I'm not a group person, more of a loner, and suddenly, sharing my deepest feelings with eight strangers wasn't easy for me. But I had to talk.

Initially, you talk more about current events because that's what's most 'alive'. The feeling you experience here and now takes precedence over underlying issues. But talking about your symptoms won't cure you; talking about what's underlying will. What suddenly struck me is that dreams suddenly became very important. Very strange ... I always thought a dream was a fantasy ... like a fairy tale or a film you watch. Certainly not something to analyse heavily. Unfortunately, I couldn't talk much about dreams myself because I hardly dreamed … or at least not that I was aware of. But otherwise, I had a lot to say. And things that seemed so self-evident had a heavier meaning than I initially thought. Slowly but surely, I worked my way to the group's top. When my therapist told me that I was the best-performing patient in the group, I felt wonderful!

Yet, I experienced challenging times during that period. Also, people who could barely speak because they were so sad affect you. The psychotherapist usually remained icily attentive. I struggled with that at the time. I could talk for three-quarters of an hour about how bad I had felt again the previous weekend, and then a little smile appeared … Awful! But when I spoke of feelings towards my mother, there was much more attention. One particular answer from the psychotherapist was the best gift I had received until then. I felt so bad that I asked, 'Will I ever get better?' He answered convincingly, 'Yes … if you continue to talk, of course.' I will never forget that; I drew much strength from it then. The individual sessions were always very enriching because then (usually at the end of the session), it was the psychiatrist who spoke, so you knew a little more about where you stood. I looked up to him enormously. If only I had had a father like that. The great absentee in my life. Someone to guide you in a man's world. There was too much mum and far too little (good) dad.

I was admitted for six months (seventeen years ago), then a year of day therapy, then weekly, and then monthly outpatient treatment until nine years ago – a hundred kilometres each way every day. I struggled with every step or change, certainly from day therapy to returning to work. I wasn't well at all. And under stress, I often felt myself withdrawing. But I succeeded, although it was a very bitter pill to swallow. A short time after returning to work, I was made redundant, and shortly afterwards, the company went bankrupt. Then, the second hell began. I still went to group therapy every Monday evening, but I was working shifts in a factory. I went deeply into the red there, or rather, I exploited my body. I had to drag myself through the day, and then I stopped group therapy as well. After that, I continued to see the psychiatrist monthly for a very long time.

What I find a bit of a misunderstanding? If you understand the cause of your suffering and go through the same process several times, you are much wiser but not cured. I never entirely became the 'old carefree K.' again. Of course, I've come a long way, but the damage and suffering were too significant to recover from fully. Then, the exploitation of my body, too much stress and too little sleep. I could study until two or three o'clock during exam week when I was still at school – five days in a row. I've never been able to do that again. One too short night, and I was/am a wreck the next day. But I can safely say that my admission did indeed save my life. I was at the end of my tether, although you couldn't tell from my outward appearance. I could hide it very well.

Looking back, I mainly find it a shame that I was born such a sensitive person. That's not a gift. Everything affects you much harder, and life weighs much heavier. That's the biggest thing for me. That's how you are, which doesn't mean you can't work on it. But you'll never become a 'hard' person. Thank God I made the right decision to get admitted at the time. Otherwise, it would undoubtedly have been fatal! It was a very long, painful, but educational process.

I want to end positively, which I'm working on now. I haven't had psychoanalysis for eight years, but I have become a father, wholly renovated my house, changed jobs (to a much better one now), and things have been going well, with ups and downs. It's a pretty good period! However, I still have a powerful bond with my mother, who is now getting older, too, and I'm increasingly preoccupied with her death. For many people, the death of a parent is a significant loss, but for me, it still means the end of the world. On top of that, I'm getting older myself, and I notice that I don't process things as well anymore. Several other ailments have also been added, including tinnitus, sleep apnoea … The first one, in particular, makes life particularly sour at times. On top of that, as a single father, I have a great responsibility for my son, and I still work full-time with on-call and evening shifts. It's challenging at times.

Ultimately, I decided to resume psychoanalysis. Unfortunately, I may have waited too long, as I recently felt like a sinking ship. I was still functioning, but I had to drag myself through the day, and I saw the future bleakly: alone, lonely, unhappy. The positive effect of years of psychotherapy was apparent but seemed so distant after all those years. Perhaps I lost sight of it due to circumstances; it's always busy, and you must move forward.

I started looking for a therapist in my area, but nothing could compare to the psychiatrist who had followed me for so long. So, after many years, I contacted him again. After a warm reunion, it was as if I had never been away. Because of the distance and his packed schedule, he sees me monthly, and on his advice, I visit a psychotherapist in my area. And honestly … what the current sessions have already achieved is remarkable! In a very short time, I already feel considerably better. I plan to continue attending sessions for a while and look forward to the future with renewed optimism. It feels good that people listen to you and try to lend a helping hand. Although there is still a taboo surrounding psychoanalysis and psychotherapy, I would advise people with mental health problems not to wait too long to seek professional help. It can be a significant turning point in your life.

19 K.V.

My journey in therapy started five years ago. I visited my GP to tell him that the stress of life was too much to bear for me. After a few appointments, he prescribes me escitalopram and refers me to a psychologist. At that point in my life, I am 25 years old. I have been depressed and suicidal, at least since my early teens. A combination of childhood trauma, growing up in an emotionless family and gender dysphoria has sent me into a downward spiral. I can't say that I ever felt genuinely normal or accepted. I feel like I have consistently hovered around the edges. Before starting therapy, I believed that my troubles had one cause. Me. Thinking that, I started on a path of self-improvement. If the problem is within me, I must have the solution. I felt like I owed it to the people around me to be the best version of myself. This was how it has always been for me. The needs of the other, or how I perceived them, had priority over mine. After years of therapy, this has somewhat lessened, but it is still there. So I started journaling, meditating, reading self-help books, practising Stoicism and Buddhism, jogging, hiking, improving my hygiene and style of clothing, trying to get out more and so on. I even changed jobs. This helped to some extent, but I needed more. After more than a year of self-improvement, I slumped again. That's how I arrived at my GP.

The psychologist I was referred to did nothing for me. She gave me the same spiel about journaling, meditation, methods of anxiety relief and other things I had tried before. She told me that she wasn't the type of psychologist who wanted me to lie down on the couch and start digging into the past. After just a few sessions, she told me she couldn't help me. I had been dishonest with her and myself about what I was feeling. These first therapy sessions were baby steps toward opening up to myself. At the end of that year, I wrote an entry in my diary asking myself if I was transgender. A few months of uselessly mulling things over passed. I decided that I could not handle this on my own, so I contacted a psychologist who specialised in questions about gender and sexuality. This is what I consider to be the proper start of my journey in therapy. It allowed me to open up, get to know myself and truly feel things. Although, that was still just the start of that process. During that period, I moved out and started living independently. I believe that the combination of not having to keep up appearances all day, beginning to open up and experimenting with drugs caused my crash. I attempted suicide. I prefer that I try to take matters into my own hands. Even after all these years, my biggest regret is not dying on that day.

This attempt led to me being hospitalised. For two months, I stayed in the psychiatric ward of a general hospital. My experience is that they do damage control and risk assessment. I was kept docile with a cocktail of anti-psychotics and antidepressants. I later heard that they refer to it as a 'reset'. The team there decided that I needed further treatment and referred me to a psychiatric hospital. After an intake appointment that felt like a police interrogation, I was assigned to 'CLIPP' – clinical psychodynamic psychotherapy.

I remember that the psychologist there called me very stoic and unreadable. I was also told that I was angry a lot. Looking back, that was true. There was a lot of hate and frustration. At the time, I just felt depressed and lonely. Surrounded by patients and staff, but still lonely.

One morning, a nurse came to my room to get me out of bed. I had much trouble motivating myself. She told me that she regretted the situation. I said that I was sorry for being such a terrible patient. She answered that she didn't regret the situation for herself but for me. I deserved so much more; it was the first time I genuinely felt cared for and someone wanted me to improve for my sake.

We had to do a few assignments when arriving at the psychiatric hospital. One of them was to tell the story of our life. Mine started with the words, 'I had a fairly normal childhood'. It was through group therapy that I dis-covered how wrong I was about this. Other patients talked about toxic beha-viour by those closest to them. I recognised my father in a lot of these stories. I started to learn about emotional abuse. What it is and what its effects are.

Delving into my past showed me how much had gone wrong. I had frequent nightmares about a surgery I had when I was three. I don't remember the surgery, but it left its traces. I bore much resentment towards my parents for that. The surgery was a simple circumcision for reasons of hygiene. This was not a valid reason. My parents brushed it off by saying that they just followed the doctor's recommendation. At the hospital, they mocked me because I had a panic attack. This happened again and again. Being mocked instead of supported. Being put down instead of being praised. Being ignored instead of stimulated.

I grew up as an empty shell. A shell that didn't even like their shell. My dad's mockery went so far that I questioned my manhood. I still wonder how that affected my gender identity.

At the hospital, the focus was on group therapy, which was split into psy-chotherapy, music therapy and expression therapy. This was further supple-mented with 'expertise' therapy, a mix of therapy, psycho-education, practical education and leisure, all tailored to the patient's needs.

In music therapy, I learned how emotions affect the body. The first time the therapist asked me 'where' I felt my sadness, I thought she had gone mad. Sadness is in the head, right? By opening up to the bodily sensations, I started to understand better what I was feeling and how to react. Years of meditation and breathing exercises have only now begun to make sense.

Both expression and music therapy taught me how much I needed to create. I have always wanted to make things and express myself through music, painting and drawing. However, my chronically low self-esteem stop-ped me from doing so. I would hate myself if I did something poorly – I genuinely detest myself. These therapies gave me a safe space in which I was encouraged to experiment.

The effect was marked. I found many things within myself that I had pushed down for years. The safety of these therapies grew into a general feeling of safety in the hospital. That allowed me to experiment with my expression as a woman.

In 'expertise' therapies, I learned about meaning in life, philosophy, mentali-sation and understanding the past. There were also more light-hearted sessions, such as improv (improvisational) theatre, gardening and group jogging.

All these insights fed back into the group and individual psychotherapy. There, I could delve deeper into the causes and effects of my feelings. The stories of other people gave me insights into my own story. I started under-standing what had happened and why. I learnt what emotional abuse is. I learnt about my parents' depression.

The practical effects of this all were not what I had hoped. Constant dig-ging into my emotions and past left me vulnerable and depressed. I had a desperate need to be cared for, and when I felt that need was not met, I attempted suicide for a second time. This was a desperate attempt for attention. It worked. Medication was increased, individual therapy was increased, and I was allowed to sleep at the hospital for a longer time than usual.

Resentment against my parents reached a boiling point. I had a massive fight with my father. We made up but walked on eggshells around each other. It took more than a year for it to start to mellow out. My relationship with my father has improved about three years after the argument. There is an unspoken agreement that we don't talk about what happened. My mother developed dementia and is slipping away. I took my parents' cat into my place because he attacked my mother.

All this makes visits to and from my parents draining, although I must say that most things in my life are draining. I had difficulty adapting at the start of the cat's life with me. I had to get out of bed for his breakfast, or he would make a ruckus. I had to clean his litterbox, or he would go on my couch. It helped get my life back on the rails.

After fourteen months in the psychiatric hospital, I returned home. I had weekly appointments with my psychologist and monthly with my psychiatrist. These were more focused on the struggles in my daily life, such as my inability to keep going to keep going to the art academy. After three months, I started working again. My low self-esteem led to stress, which lowered my performance and thus validated my low self-esteem. A secondary frustration was that both my psychologist and psychiatrist tried to tell me it was all in my head. I was doing poorly at work – enough to get not one but two negative evaluations.

I managed to hold on because I had a trip to Vietnam to look forward to. When I got back from the trip, I spent a miserable day at home, then went to the emergency room to get re-admitted to the psychiatry ward. A few days later, I was fired for my poor performance. About a month later, I was admitted to the same psychiatric hospital that I had previously spent fourteen months in.

I can honestly say that the year and three months outside of the hospital gave me enormous insight into what I needed to function like a 'normal' person. I got a new piercing, and my first tattoo, shaved my hair again, and I genuinely started to love myself. For the first time, I didn't hate the person I saw in the mirror.

Music and expression therapy were instrumental towards this change. Being able to exchange something that runs deeper than words. It also meant that I didn't need words for everything anymore. In that light, I think the closest word for my gender now is non-binary. I would describe it as it is what it is. I can finally see what I want and do what I want without overthinking it constantly. My head remains a war zone of competing analyses of every tiny thing I do and like. I think it used to be *twelve angry men* playing at quadruple speed. But now it has calmed down to just *twelve angry men.*

Anxiety and a certain degree of mental anguish remain my loyal companions. I still have trouble motivating myself to leave my house. I still use antipsychotics to find some modicum of rest in my head. Overall, I think I have not improved as a person. I have become an actual person. I evolved from an empty husk to a psychiatric patient to being myself. Finally, I have formed an identity that is more than a shallow reflection of the situation around me.

20 M.C.

In my mid-thirties, I crashed. I worked a lot, earned well and literally and figuratively flew from pillar to post, but I wasn't happy. I couldn't see a way out; a desperate act seemed the only escape.

Looking back, I had little understanding of what was going on. I was stuck in an unrequited love for a straight man. I felt rejected, hurt, not good enough and so on. I was also, in a way, living a double life. I always presented a 'nice façade'. I like to surround myself with nice things. I find that important. Presenting myself well is also crucial for my self-esteem. I've always been like that. Perhaps I picked it up from home?

Despite the many troubles, arguments and tensions at home (because of my alcoholic father), Mum always carried on, and my older brother and I followed her example. Back then, our house was surrounded by a high (perfectly trimmed) hedge, but much misery was hidden behind that hedge. Mum essentially kept things together, and nothing was discussed outwardly. We were good children who obeyed. Even after another sleepless night (my father could rage for hours on end when he came home drunk), we'd go to school the following day without a word ... Nobody noticed or said anything ...

But behind the façade, a sad heap of misery was hidden. Still, I couldn't quite grasp it. Therapy made it clear how important a loving mother and father are. It also became clear that I had 'too much' mother and far too little father. A father who protects you but also sets boundaries. My father deserves much recognition because he was a master in woodwork. He could make absolutely anything out of wood. From the most considerable renovation to what seemed technically impossible, he could do it. But as a child, I couldn't appreciate that. When he'd been drinking, he transformed into a monster. How can a child cope with such duality? Who is your father? The negative far outweighed his positive sides (which he did have).

As a child, I also couldn't rebel against my father. When he was sober, I pretty much got everything I wanted ... (even if I didn't get it from Mum). So, you learn quickly as a child to get what you want. Somewhere, I tried to move forward; I wanted to stand rapidly on my two feet. To earn money to buy what I wanted (to compensate for what I unconsciously missed and couldn't buy ...).

I was bullied at school quite early on. I was too good ... From about the age of twelve, I struggled with authority. I changed schools on average every two years.

When I was fifteen, I went to a real boys' boarding school where I didn't find my place. I didn't count, so I got into things to get noticed. As always, I had to figure things out for myself.

I lent money to pupils who didn't get any (or enough) from home and got it back the following week with interest. I also sometimes sold some of my clothes.

After the boys' boarding school, I ended up in a dorm and attended a girls' school that had just become mixed (there were three boys amongst twenty-two girls). But even there, I didn't find my place. I struggled enormously with my sexuality. I was pretty popular with the girls but didn't know what to do with it, so I spent much time – feeling very lonely – in my room. That's where the first suicidal thoughts surfaced. My landlady was a real mother to me, and I was her favourite. She cooked for me every day. To ease my inner suffering, and because I had no friends, I'd go to Knokke (in Belgium) on free afternoons to buy clothes.

As an adolescent, I'd had a few consultations with a psychiatrist, but it didn't amount to anything beyond being prescribed some antidepressants. When I collapsed, I went to see my GP, and he was the catalyst for a new beginning. He took the time to listen and offered me three options. First, I want to go ahead with what I planned. Second, to start medication and try to carry on (with outpatient therapy). Third, to start medication and begin intensive support (admission for clinical psychotherapy). He favoured the third option. After discussions with some family members and friends, I agreed to an intake interview with an assistant psychiatrist. Shortly afterwards, I was admitted for six months of full-time inpatient treatment, followed by three months of day therapy.

This all seems to have gone smoothly (technically, it did), but psychologically, it was a massive step for me. I remember feeling entirely like a failure; I saw no way out, but I also didn't know what to expect from admission or whether it would even help my hopeless situation. So, I didn't have any immediate expectations, but I had to trust the good intentions of my GP, who fully supported the admission. It was sink or swim …

During my admission, there was group psychotherapy three times a week. Although this can be (very) difficult at times for a layman (and/or a shy person), I'm convinced it works for most people. Hearing other people's stories, recognising and acknowledging. This was supplemented by a weekly or bi-weekly individual session with the psychiatrist and/or psychologist. Things that came up during group therapy and other therapies could be discussed more deeply in a personal session.

It isn't easy to pinpoint precisely what helped. It's a combination of several things. Being (temporarily) removed from society, away from everything, only having to focus on yourself and your process, the combination of different therapies, the support of the various healthcare professionals (who are well-informed about the patient's progress), etc. It's also essential that the patient is consciously or unconsciously willing to work on themselves. To be (willing to) open (themselves) up… I particularly remember the psycho-education 'I was a CPMP child' as being very valuable for me specifically.

I grew up with an alcohol-abusing father. Because of his physical violence, this caused a lot of tension and insecurity. We had to flee our home several times. The threats and tensions were mainly psychological. When my father had been drinking, he could shout, yell, and rant incessantly for hours. He threw doors, cupboards, and chairs, but I don't directly remember physical violence. The threat of it, yes.

I didn't let myself be pushed around and challenged by my father. I shouted back (when I was older), while my older brother was more of a peacemaker. He tried to reason with my father and calm him down. When we were very young, Mum had to protect us and sometimes chose to flee (to her parents or sister).

Out of shame and a preference for keeping her relationship problems 'in-house', this remained very limited. We often fled to a room where we locked ourselves while Father hammered on the door. Sometimes, Mum called the police, locking my father up for a night. Or worse, they would come, say a few calming words, and then leave. Of course, this was like fueling the fire, and Father became a raging bull.

When we got older, we had to protect each other. My father was, to the outside world, the most exemplary man. Always ready to help someone, he was indeed the devil to his family in the cruellest sense of the word when drunk.

I also found the expressive therapy forum very insightful. This therapy was unknown to me. You might think, what's the point of making a drawing? But I was shocked at how certain things came to the surface in this way and taught/told you something about yourself – for example, the task of drawing a house. I drew a beautiful, large home and worked out in detail: an attractive façade, driveway, planting, etc. I don't remember exactly, but you had to draw yourself and your parents somewhere. But the most striking thing for me was to fill the house and make the interior layout. I remember that I was utterly blocked here. I couldn't get that inside 'in order'. It tells how I felt/was at the time – a 'polished' exterior with an empty interior. The reference to the home situation could also be made in this way, I think... I also remember that during my admission, I never walked around in pyjamas or tracksuits. No matter how bad I felt, I would never leave my room like that!

I can't immediately name anything that wouldn't have helped. All the tools provided contributed to the process to a greater or lesser extent. Even things that, at first glance, don't contribute can say something or bring something to the surface as to why they wouldn't help.

Roughly speaking, my psychotherapeutic process lasted ten years. After discharge, I gradually returned to work with outpatient psychotherapy. Weekly for the first few years, then gradually from bi-weekly to monthly. I think that once you start a psychotherapeutic process, you can't/can never consider it 'finished'. Life goes on with expected and unexpected events/set-backs, and you don't always know in advance how you'll react to them. The skill is to use what you have learned and gained from your process to cope with this resilience. It's also the art of allowing yourself a lousy day because being 'unhappy' occasionally is also part of life. Of course, you must also be aware of pitfalls that can quickly lead you back into a downward spiral.

I can't say whether there are good or bad therapists. One (approach of a) therapist works better or worse for different patients.

Overall, I look back with positive feelings. Without support, there was a high chance I wouldn't be here today. The therapy (and medication) helped me become calmer and more resilient. It also helped me see specific insights and connections that I wouldn't have been able to see without therapy. Looking ahead, it's not a bad idea to keep a line open between therapist and patient.

21 M.D.B.

When I started psychotherapy, I had no realistic picture of my childhood. I built a fantasy world to survive. As a child, I often invented how fantastic it was at home. My view now is much more realistic but also much more painful.

When I was in my mid-twenties, I consulted my psychiatrist at a psychiatric hospital. At first glance, I was an ordinary twenty-something; I had a three-year relationship with a great guy, had graduated with honours from university with a degree in physiotherapy, and worked in both a group practice and my practice. But I wasn't happy; I suffered from severe anxiety attacks and depression and had already overcome an eating disorder. In short, things weren't going well at all.

By telling my story, I discovered that the family I grew up in wasn't a typical middle-class family. There was little warmth, cosiness and love. Even more, there was a lot of aggression, threat and hopelessness. The ingredients for growing into a well-adjusted adult who feels good about themselves and believes in a positive future were missing.

Meanwhile, I know that my problems started in my early years. There are serious deficiencies in my relationship with my mother. I never had a close bond with her, which made me feel very lonely. She is a narcissistic and selfish woman who is jealous of her daughters. I had a slightly warmer relationship with my father, but he had many 'issues', which meant I couldn't turn to him either. He was often depressed, aggressive and transgressive, making it very unsafe to grow up near him, let alone become a woman.

Until I was eight, I found a lot of comfort and love in my best friend's family. I was a regular visitor and tried to be there as often as possible. When my parents came to pick me up after a sleepover, I would hide because I didn't want to go home at all.

Despite everything, I was a cheerful child. I enjoyed school, had many friends, played tennis and piano, and took dance lessons. Unfortunately, my parents decided to move when I was eight, and the loss of my familiar school and environment and my friend's family made my problems much worse. I changed from a cheerful child into a quiet, shy and unhappy girl. I was no longer the outgoing one. I refused to continue my hobbies; I slowly faded away.

Around twelve, I started fantasising about my parents and sister being better off without me. I started blaming myself for our 'unhappy family'. This is when my suicidal thoughts began. Shortly afterwards, my father became terminally ill and died when I was fifteen. This is the first time I remember being genuinely depressed. I went to a psychiatrist for the first time but dropped out.

Studying at university kept me going; I drew strength from my studies! After my studies, I decided to seek help again. That's how I ended up with my psychiatrist. For me, the admission was a relief. Finally, there was someone who listened to me. Finally, I could discover who I was in a safe environment – finally, someone who understood me. Finally, some people believed in me. Finally, I could remove my mask and show what was hidden behind it. Finally, I could catch up on some of my missed childhood, adolescence and young adulthood. Finally, a future?

When I started psychotherapy, I had no idea of the seriousness of my problems. First, I never thought an analysis would take years. Second, I was always convinced that the more I talked, the more my problems would melt away like snow in the sun. Just as I threw myself into my studies at university, I did everything I could to make my psychotherapeutic process successful – and it was a great success.

It was a disappointment to realise that it doesn't work like that. Unfortunately, I can't erase my early years, and psychotherapy doesn't give me immunity from further adversity in life. But psychotherapy has been my salvation; that much is certain. I dare say I wouldn't be here without psychotherapeutic help!

The therapy has given me insights that have changed not only my thinking but also my actions. Of course, this didn't happen overnight; after all, I had been living/suffering for a long time in a way that didn't make me happy … You don't change that lifestyle overnight.

What changes have I noticed in myself? I'm still the same person but more confident in my private and professional life. I love myself more. I take better care of myself. I'm kinder to myself. I give myself compliments regularly. I try not to set the bar so high. I no longer blame myself. I learned that life doesn't have to be like it used to be; it can be different. I try to look at myself through different glasses than my parents used to look at me. I now understand why I ended up in a depression. I realise I can't replace my mother and father with a new and better model, but I can try to be a good mother and father to myself!

Several things played an essential role in my recovery. Let me list a few … Every week, I look forward to Friday's cooking activity with D.! We cooked in a homely atmosphere and then ate our creations together. I learned to cook there, and this gave my self-confidence a boost. D. was a surrogate mother to me. I learned many household things from her. For the first time, I realised the importance of a family meal, how pleasant it can be to eat together, and how essential good food is for your mental and physical health. D.'s cookbook is in my kitchen cupboard. To this day, I enjoy the fruits of her labour with my husband and friends.

There was a creative workshop in the heart of the ward where I was admitted. I spent hours under the watchful eye of G. Painting, dyeing, sculpting, drawing, etc. Today, I know that creativity is healing. I regularly immerse myself in a bath of creative activity.

I often felt alone in the world, unconnected to anything or anyone. My admission allowed me to build relationships with therapists that remained intact despite disagreements or conflicts. This is how my trust in people gradually grew, how I dared to confront conflicts and how my self-belief grew.

During my admission, my eyes were opened to so many people with mental health problems. During the group sessions, you get support from fellow patients. Fellow patients telling their stories help you to come forward with your own story.

My psychiatrist often talks about Mother P. (the name of the psychiatric hospital). The ward where I was admitted had a very homely feel. Therapists and patients usually sat together in the living room between therapy sessions. They talked, laughed, knitted, played board games, read, etc. I enjoyed this pleasant togetherness and the security and safety surrounding it.

My psychotherapeutic process took about fifteen years. During this period, I alternated residential admissions, day therapy and outpatient therapy. During admissions and day therapy, I worked full-time on myself. During outpatient therapy, I practised my profession and took significant steps forward, such as finding a home, a garden and a tree.

I can only touch on a few things. I have a love/hate relationship with toy shops. On the one hand, I would like to buy everything my child's heart desires; on the other hand, I want to run away from them. Disney films, comics, books, fairy tales, bedtime stories, Lego, colouring books, craft materials … were alien to me. I had one Tintin comic, one Lego house, and one Barbie doll. To be clear, I didn't grow up in poverty; my parents had the means.

Shopping is a real ordeal for me! Yet I love beautiful and well-dressed people. I love fabrics and clothes with gorgeous cuts. This phobia is a leftover from shopping with my mother. In the shop, her true nature came to the surface. I didn't get the clothes and shoes I liked; my clothes weren't bought in the correct size; there was always an argument between her and the shop assistants about the correct size. She messed with the prices of the clothes, constantly haggled for a discount, pulled all the clothes off the shelves, and bought the clothes I liked for herself. I thought I had a shoe size different from my actual shoe size for years.

All this caused me such stress and shame that, at a certain point, I no longer wanted to shop. Later, when I had my first bit of money, I bought something I liked. I hid it in my wardrobe, and when my mother wasn't home, I would put it on in my room. That was my moment of happiness.

I never felt safe at home. My parents would come into my room unexpectedly all the time – my bedroom, the bathroom, the toilet, even when I was menstruating. My father threw a tissue in the toilet whenever I was in the bathroom. The bathroom was a nightmare for me. Inappropriately, comments about my body from both of them were commonplace. Constant commentary on everything – the way I washed my face, the amount of water I used, remarks about my breasts. The same horror every morning.

My day hadn't started, and I was already completely wound up. The looks from both of them still give me chills to this day. From her, it was more jealousy of my body; from him, it was transgressive and sexist. I never had any privacy. My body was more theirs than mine.

I remember the first time I got my period. I was barely eleven; my father laughed at me in a way that made me shudder. My mother gave me the necessary sanitary towels without more. Because of this, I developed shame about my body.

The desolate feeling I've had since I was a baby can still surface. I feel abandoned very quickly. Nightmares about the past come and go. Insecurity lurks around the corner. I search for mothers and potential mother figures in my professional and personal life. Trusting someone and building a bond with someone remains a real challenge for me! Feeling like a beautiful woman and allowing myself to be attractive remains a daily task.

I detest my parents for the way they treated me. A bitterness has settled deep within me. I'm angry at everything and everyone around me. I am angry because I didn't have a happy childhood. I was angry because they could have spared me much suffering. I was angry because my mother didn't give me any love. I was angry because they didn't think I was worthwhile. Angry about that invisible pain that often leaves you alone with it. Angry about talking until you're hoarse. Angry about the missed opportunities. I was angry because I wasn't allowed to become/be a woman. Angry because they broke me instead of making me. Sometimes, I want to shout it from the rooftops! *HELP! I'M IN NEED! I'M HURT! I'M WOUNDED! CAN'T YOU SEE THIS?* In the past, the anger was sometimes so bad that suicide seemed the only way out. Fortunately, I've learned that talking about that anger helps.

I was never abused in the literal sense of the word. Yet I feel abused to the very core of my being! During group sessions, I discovered that I show similar symptoms to people who have been abused. In a public toilet or at people's homes, I hold the doorknob with one hand, fearing that someone will come in. After exercising, I always shower at home. When we go on holiday with friends, I find sharing the bathroom and toilet difficult. If our neighbours invite me for a swim, I decline. Going to the beach in a bikini with friends is a challenge. When I had brain surgery, my biggest fear was the catheter during general anaesthesia. During our fertility treatment, I had to constantly remind myself that all those examinations and looks from the doctors were necessary to help us have a baby.

Meanwhile, I have a warm, safe and pleasant home with my husband. I can say that I have found true love! He is my great love, partner and best friend; we are a top team in good times and bad.

With him by my side, I see a future. I have a job I'm proud of. I now work at a maternity ward where we support young parents. Those days, months and the first year are so crucial. Love that is so crucial in a human life. Most parents are in love with their baby. Unconditional love! That's how it should be!

And what about the future? I'm in a grieving process. My husband and I would have loved to have a family where love would be central. Meanwhile, I know better than anyone what a child needs to grow into a full version of themselves, ready to face the cruel world. We've been through a long, fruitless process. Mother Nature decided otherwise ...

Because of this grieving process, I now go to see my psychiatrist twice a week. This setback affects me very deeply, so much so that sometimes I feel like I'm right back at the beginning of my process. And yet, deep down, I know it will be all right. *Andrà tutto bene!* (Everything will be okay!).

And yet, the spirits in my head remain. And I realise they will always be there. They are a part of me. And this despite years of psychotherapy, the unconditional love of my husband, the presence of friends and the few family members I have. But I now have a more realistic picture of what has been. Because that's what psychotherapy does; it doesn't erase it, but it gives insight, softens things and puts things in perspective, making it all a bit easier to bear.

22 M.D.M.

I was married to my childhood sweetheart, had two children and had a good job. My life was running smoothly; I seemingly had it all together. I was the type to tackle things and persevere, and I could juggle many things simultaneously. Nothing quickly overwhelmed me. I was a busy bee both at home and at work. Hard work and control were necessary. I felt responsible for many people and issues but unconsciously neglected my health. There was no indication that I would experience mental health problems. Until the day my daughter became a victim of sexual abuse ...

Initially, I held it together. I was ready to support her. However, my comforting words angered her. She felt I didn't understand her. The situation triggered my drive for perfection to alleviate the painful emotions. It forced me to do more. Try harder. Achieve more. Every attempt to show understanding and comfort only confirmed the opposite. I proved incapable of helping my daughter; my maternal instinct hit an unprecedented limit. I was in such pain, such grief for her. It was everywhere – in my head, heart, and whole body. I felt myself slipping away. Life turned black.

That mental state caused concentration problems and memory loss. The worrying also made it difficult to sleep; I woke up early in the morning and would lie there worrying about the day ahead. I would burst into tears unexpectedly and felt irritable quickly. I could no longer relax. I channelled my restlessness into an overactive work ethic at work, but at home I felt exhausted. I was stuck in a mire and fighting a war against myself. Nothing in my behaviour or thoughts resembled the person I used to be.

My GP was both concerned and decisive. Admission to the hospital for treatment was necessary. I stayed at the PWGH (in the psychiatric acute admission unit) for three weeks, mainly to rest. Then, I was admitted to a clinical psychotherapeutic ward of a psychiatric hospital. There, I could address the underlying causes that had led me there: my excessive caring, perfectionism, difficulty saying no, etc.

The admission was intense, painful and revealing. It completely overwhelmed me. The psychiatrist's approach also made me doubt. I wanted a diagnosis, treatment and a clear path to recovery. It needed to be predictable and preferably time limited. The timeframe was indefinite. The doctor didn't think a diagnosis would be beneficial for me. According to him, I was 'overwrought'. I concluded that my situation wasn't serious. Was that why I had abandoned my family and work?

During the intake interview, the psychiatrist also pointed out that my husband was my first and only love. He asked if I had seen a father figure in him. I felt insulted, as if, like a little child, I had been looking for a daddy instead of a partner. Throughout the process, I realised he was right. I had indeed sought a lover with qualities I missed in my father – a man who could protect me and whom I could trust.

I underwent a deluge of therapy: psychotherapy, creative therapy, music therapy, process facilitation, verbal communication, sports … Weeks of confrontations, crying, loneliness and support followed. I had to get used to the way of working. I didn't always understand why things were expected of me. Playing my favourite sport, badminton, seemed pointless until I realised how much anger I had when I hit the shuttlecock hard. I found the group sessions very difficult. I took other people's problems away from the sessions without resolving my own. It even led to a conflict when a woman with an addiction history described how miserable she felt because her children didn't like her. 'How could those children like an addict?' I wondered.

My father also had an alcohol problem. I preferred not to bring friends home because I was ashamed of his behaviour. I have no good memories of my father. No moments of joy, no pats on the back, no hugs. I feel he never really liked me. I empathised with the woman's children and vented my frustrations on her during the session.

The first night, I shared a room with two young people. I knew that one of them exhibited self-harming behaviour. I lay anxiously listening to all sorts of unfamiliar noises when I suddenly thought the girl was cutting or scratching herself. My maternal instinct tried to fight against my fear. What if she hurt herself so badly that she bled to death? What should I do? I shivered in my bed and hardly dared to move. I felt responsible for her. When the night nurse came by, and I quietly told her, she said: 'You don't need to worry about it; she's just putting on an act. It's her way of seeking attention.' I was stunned by her response. Where had I ended up? Weren't we taken seriously here? Was I also putting on an act? Her reaction brought me even lower. I wanted to switch to day therapy as soon as possible.

After a week, I got a single room where I was content with my company. I felt better. Still, I longed for home. I was relieved to get the psychiatrist's approval; thanks to the strong support of my family, I was able to switch to day therapy after one month of inpatient treatment. Six months later, this transitioned into years of outpatient therapy. I was relieved but also scared of the hectic life I would return to. Of that real life outside the clinic with all the pressure and stimuli. It was a learning process to prepare myself for that.

During my admission, I reacted to intense confrontations by running away. The turmoil inside me gave me the feeling, the urge, a reflex to want to be somewhere else. I fled, thinking I could escape the unrest. I wanted to leave the hospital, so I went outside and kept walking. Hours later, I returned with a small, frightened heart. 'Me, a mother of two teenagers running away, you can't justify that,' I thought. The nurses reacted sympathetically. Their first aim was to unblock the crisis and stress situation by talking to me and finding out what had triggered me.

In therapy, you're dependent in a certain way; you open yourself up to a stranger. For a long time, I saw the psychiatrist like my supervisor at work; as a strict father to whom I mainly wanted to tell what was going well. I had to get used to him sitting silently and expressionlessly, staring ahead and occasionally asking: 'What does that remind you of? Why do you think that is? ...'. I couldn't bear the silences he allowed. It took a while before I clicked with him. At those moments, all sorts of thoughts came up: 'What does he think of me now? He must think I'm stupid.' I still longed for a quick, tangible transformation. I wanted to see the results of my efforts. It frustrated me that repressed memories had such an impact on me that after a session, I felt further away from recovery than before.

The therapist doesn't provide answers or solutions; he helps you find them yourself. Only after several years of therapy did I realise the value of this method. You also remember the answer to a riddle longer if you found the solution yourself. This realisation was stimulating and healing. At certain moments, I felt that the psychologist and the psychiatrist were challenging me, that they knew the solution but deliberately withheld it from me. The request to speak openly, without censorship, was complex.

In the first stage of my process, resistance prevented me from getting to the essence, and I talked endlessly about trivial things or said nothing for a long time, although my head was bubbling with anger. I didn't want to say anything. Afterwards, I was angry and disappointed with myself for having wasted an opportunity (session).

It takes an enormous effort to talk about your thoughts and feelings without a filter – an effort where you don't spare yourself. You push hard on sore spots and have to trust that the pain will lessen, provided you allow it. I often avoided the psychiatrist's gaze; it helped me dig deep into my past without losing myself too quickly emotionally.

I also needed time to embrace the help of the psychiatrist and psychologist. They didn't shy away from difficult situations; their approach was straightforward, without any fuss. A strategy that suits me very well. Trust grew steadily but became strong enough to withstand conflicts. Conflicts rooted in my most profound turmoil, which I only dared to express through them. Today, the psychiatrist is the only person who truly knows me. He helped me reconstruct my story and find solutions. Even after completing the therapy, he remains my anchor point. If things ever worsen, I won't hesitate to contact him.

If they had told me that outpatient therapy would last ten years, I would have given up. Now, I'm proud that I persevered and discovered what burdens were dragging me down. Although the confrontation sometimes plunged me even deeper. Knowing the triggers doesn't remove them. Learning to cope with them is a grieving process, and the danger of everything overwhelming you again never completely disappears.

I thought I knew myself well, but everything was turned upside down. I discovered things in myself that I didn't want to see. During a consultation, I sometimes felt so emotionally overwhelmed that I got up and ran away like a child. The frozen anger thawed, and I exploded. Flashbacks overwhelmed me, and I had to show and vent my anger. Because of my daughter's court case, I directed my anger at the police. I drove recklessly; fines didn't bother me. I challenged them by moving into their bumper and shouted at them when they noticed I was parked incorrectly.

The initial referral due to my daughter's trauma was quickly supplemented by my 'own stuff'. I was carrying so much. I didn't find safety and security in my parents' home – instead, I was in an unstable situation. I learned early to adapt my behaviour to others, so I constantly walked on eggshells. For a long time, I also believed I wasn't clever and didn't amount to much. I felt strongly inferior because I didn't get the chance to further my education. During training and exams at work, I had a fear of failure. I discovered the root cause of this low self-esteem.

I discovered mountains of pent-up anger that go back to my childhood. As a child, reproaches, criticism, comments, orders and threats were thrown at me. I learned to cope with this by installing behaviour patterns that characterised me as an adult. I would do anything to avoid anyone being disappointed in me. I knew no limits in this and didn't consider myself; the craving for love was too intense.

The sessions catapulted me back to my childhood, and after months of talking, I had to discover that I was a grown-up teenager. I had skipped my adolescence. My whole self was built on shifting sand: an unfinished foundation. I had to go back to that foundation, to that adolescence. Only when I finished that could I slowly start rebuilding everything, this time without the construction errors of then. I relived my past and started behaving like that, too, both towards the psychiatrist and at home. I constantly wanted to sit on my husband's lap, asked him to spoon me in bed, and behaved childishly.

The years after the admission were also challenging. The world kept turning, and the memories of the past greatly impacted how I dealt with the present. After my father's death, a stupid question provoked a violent reaction from my mother. She slammed down the phone, came towards me, and started yelling. She angered me so much that I decided to break contact with her. That wasn't easy, and an inner struggle preceded it. Moreover, you encounter many misunderstandings when you break up with your parents.

The break-up took up a large part of the therapeutic process. A break-up that seemed irreparable. I didn't want to see her again, ever. Staying in contact caused too much pain. I avoided her and cut myself from the whole family, including my younger brother and sister. I thought the break-up would bring peace. It didn't lead to relief; it gave me the feeling of being lost and unfree. I missed her. There was always a space at the table on birthdays, Christmas, and Mother's Day, and I couldn't fully enjoy it. When I underwent some major surgeries, and she knew, she sent my husband a text message wishing me well. Secretly, I hoped for a visit … This didn't happen.

Unlike my treating doctor, I didn't believe in reconciliation. I often reproached the psychiatrist for taking my mother's side because he suggested sending a card or a message. Then I was furious with him! He thought that if she were no longer there, the pain would be even more significant. I claimed the opposite, and the discussion had begun … Several times, I dreamt of visiting her. I usually woke up with a confusing feeling. What was I supposed to do with that? The doctor persisted and replied: 'If you have that feeling, you should visit her. It's the only way to find a solution.'

My husband and children were hesitant and worried. They were afraid that if it failed, it would cause me too much pain again, to which I told them that the missing also hurt. During the therapeutic process, I felt myself growing and becoming mentally stronger. It gave me energy and motivated me to seek rapprochement as the next step in my recovery. I called her and asked tremblingly if I could come over. She enthusiastically replied, 'Yes, and when?' Crying, I stammered, 'Tonight.'

The road was arduous and erratic but worthwhile. In retrospect, I consider the therapy a gift to myself. I have received recognition for the pain I suffered as a child. I have gained insight into how this pain works through my reactions to myself and others. The pain points aren't gone. News reports about sexual abuse trigger my anger; stories about 'a warm home' make me jealous. I know this and how to protect myself against it, or at least how to recover from it. I found the courage to see myself as someone who makes mistakes and is simultaneously good enough. I have become stronger as a person, I can handle more, and I am kinder to those around me. Therapy has made me a more open and fragile person. I dare to be more vulnerable because I know that achieves more than building walls. I'm not perfect, and that's okay. I even think it's better that way!

The clinic, psychiatrist and psychologist changed my life. Above all, it was a period of introspection. I incorporated more pauses and added different accents to my life. There is a balance in my physical, mental and emotional health.

These testimonials hopefully dismantle shame and offer comfort. Our society has too little ear for that. I want to end with these words from the Gnostic Gospel of Thomas: 'If you do not bring forth that which is within you, that which you do not bring forth will destroy you.'

23 M.D.P.

The first draft of this testament was a furious outburst. It is well written, easily readable and as compelling as I can write. However, the content was never fit for publication. Thankfully, there's professional confidentiality, isn't there? Vengeful cries for help might warrant thorough psychoanalysis, but it does not reflect rational thought. It certainly doesn't accurately represent the therapeutic journey my psychiatrist and psychotherapist have been providing me with for years.

I resist the urge to send him my murderous, brooding helplessness. Something I could never manage before. Today, I can create enough distance to try to put the brakes on that destructive whirlwind in my head. Brake. Rest. Brake. Rest. Until exhaustion or rationality returns, whichever comes first.

That very first restart took two years. Despite – or perhaps because of – becoming a new father, I was sleeping in the psychiatric hospital, P. 'P. is a madhouse, don't you know. They're all raving mad in there, don't you know.' My whirlwind was melodic on arrival. I was stark raving mad, and I was the one doing the driving instead of – walking.

As the first electric wheelchair user on the clinical psychotherapeutic ward, this initially caused some apprehension among the nurses. They preferred psychiatric nursing. They feared that my physical needs would overload the system. Luckily, during the waiting period before admission, I had a weekly appointment at the mental health service because the fear that I wouldn't get help due to my disability was real. They would schedule a home visit to assess me, which I refused. Ultimately, I forced my admission simply by showing up for my appointment and not leaving. A hospital bed was arranged. I had brought a hoist from home, and that was sorted.

The lengthy clinical psychotherapeutic admission is one of the most valuable periods of my life. The mix of personalities among patients and staff created a breeding ground where I could finally learn social interaction. I was pretty sociable and a joker in the past, but I never talked about myself. There was no 'me'; I only had the role of social. This led to many wonderful moments, but I never spoke about the multiple gaps within myself.

Reassembling your identity after trauma has shattered it takes time. A whole, whole, whole lot of time. The process isn't so much about rebuilding after an earthquake but about a phoenix rising again and again from its ashes. Psychiatric nursing is about sweeping those ashes together in the hope that the spark of life will re-ignite. Unfortunately, sweeping with a coarse brush doesn't work. It takes much energy, and you still have ashes left. There's no chance that phoenix will take flight. However, the multitude of techniques the psychiatrist unleashed on me was gentle enough to sweep together the heap of misery I had become. Sometimes, they stirred me gently. Sometimes, they gave me a good telling-off. Sometimes, they gave me a giant brush and told me to use it myself. Ultimately, a phoenix is nothing if it never spreads its wings.

The advantages and disadvantages of each therapy would take us too far. This is a personal feeling, anyway. One person sees a perpetrator figure in a well-meaning caregiver and turns them into monsters. Another person sees someone who genuinely wants to listen in that same caregiver. When I stopped self-harming, it was because I chose to, not because my doctor had

forbidden me. I don't know if this approach works for everyone; I only stopped self-harming when I could, not before.

The programme imposed on you isn't 'rest'. I get the creeps from PWGH
(psychiatric acute admission unit) programmes where you rest. Take pills and
carry on. It is as if igniting your personality only requires lying down. Ultimately, I have a doctor who, from day one, acknowledged that I had a personality. The more I try to build a dialectic with people, the more I notice
how lucky I've been. The stereotypes people fall back on when they see
someone 'different' also translate into how you address people in that different way. He only called me by my first name.

The individual counsellor there, the person who taught me to use clay, the
music therapist, that cleaner in the corridor, those initially hated and later so
sorely missed nurses, that fellow patient and now friend whom I often see
again, and the many beautiful, handwritten cards I received when I said
goodbye to everyone I knew – the tearful outburst of gratitude. The container
is full of visual art. I don't know if these elements are what made me rise
again. But suddenly, I can never start again when I've planned it, never when
it's convenient. Only when I can start again after I've burned out.

Ultimately, two years, eight of which were mainly spent asleep, was a relatively short period that greatly impacted my current personality. I have a
pottery room. The clay gives me a sense of calm, and my figurative creations
always represent a piece of the shattered puzzle that I am. Often, they are
dark pieces. I find it difficult to sculpt the light-coloured pieces. They feel
forced, as if they're going to disrupt my composition. There's a figurine of
me – unfinished – waiting until I can start working on it again.

Without the process of therapy, expression, socialisation, psycho-education
and a thousand cups of coffee from those rancid coffee machines, I would
never have managed to turn the self-hatred and mistrust I slowly felt on arrival at the psychiatric hospital into lasting care for my loved ones. Through
the outbursts of anger, which my wife also shares in, there appears to be a
strong fabric of a material I can't quite place. It's supportive yet flexible,
warm and supportive. Love? My therapist calls it 'normal'.

My psychiatrist has become used to my outbursts of anger. How blind he is to
the reality that nobody understands me, indeed not my therapist! His great for-
tune is that I rarely explode in his office. Only via email. Not that he hasn't got
tired of reading them, the same accusation every time. Fighting windmills, but
what if you are the windmill yourself? Yet he continues to read, to respond, to
translate insights. Not only mine but his own, and that's brilliant. He is genuinely
fond of his patients. The safety of a computer screen is lacking with my psychotherapist, where I had an outburst of anger in her office twice a week. A
wheelchair user can't kick anyone, but I can damn well retaliate verbally.

My psychotherapist is terrific. Not just because she's kind and skilled but
mainly because she still hasn't chewed me out and or abandoned me. Even
when everyone else would give up, the door always opens again. Everything

my mother should have heard, she's taken. In between, she listened, offered confirmation and raised her own family. Every time a new member joined, I felt excluded and abused her. Until the whirlwind stopped again when she replied to my email; she was terrific. But in the morning, I wake up furious and beg the psychiatrist to change therapists because there's no progress. It's just that you can't choose your patients …

I don't need to say sorry. Therapy hurts. I am experiencing growing pains. While I am grateful to my psychiatrist and my psychotherapist for their determination, I must also acknowledge my role. The whirlwind is there. Despite all those doubts and fears of abandonment, I continue to trust her and my psychiatrist's judgement. I'm persevering, too. If someone reading this finds this evident, they must have grown slower than I did.

I managed to get my diploma in further education. I carried my teddy bear with me everywhere. When I lost sight of it on the way, some of my classmates wanted to organise a poster campaign. I am very grateful to my fellow students for their genuine friendship.

It's a shame that I completed the entire course in a year. I was in a hurry. I took the next step as rashly as my decision to graduate. University. I may have chosen psychology, but I was afraid that once I understood the therapist's tricks, I would also unravel my recovery. Someone who had spent a lifetime in the 'armchair' and was now reflecting on life, I chose philosophy. I discovered that I am the only type of philosopher the professor didn't elaborate on: the critic. You mustn't leave a single question unanswered.

University was, admittedly, mainly to prove to my mother that I didn't have a mental disability. I posted the results of my exams on Facebook because I knew it was the only way to get her attention. She liked it. My father, who is somewhere in the Philippines surrounded by 'chickens and rabbits' – according to his second of three emails in the last two decades – also liked it. He recently contacted me through my mother. I refused.

Also, like all students, I wanted to travel by train and then by bike. This effort required enormous planning, leaving my family with hardly any time with me. I discovered a new social struggle. Ableism: discrimination against people with disabilities. With a wheelchair, I must compulsorily book a train ticket daily. Or there's nowhere to find a toilet, certainly not where toilets are for 'normal' people. Now that the coronavirus crisis has made it clear to people what it means mentally to stand at doors you want to go through but can't, I hope we're #woke about how this remains the norm for every wheelchair user.

I first experienced this #crip activism in the inaccessibility of the university, about which I have since delighted the vice-chancellor with a presentation. It's been heard that it needs to improve, but I'm going further: first, I need a focus group. I will study law at the same university in September by taxi. I am within my rights.

Meanwhile, the relationship between my mother and me is re-established. There was an outburst of anger towards my mother – about using the doorbell – and a day later, we calmly talked things through. Plans have been discussed, and a loving arrangement has been worked out, equally divided to the penny between my brother and myself. She can supplement her pension, my brother can rebuild his life after the relationship breakdown, and I can move if I want to.

My mother does much more for me than my father ever did. But she constantly seeks conflict-free situations. Within her relationships, there is never conflict. She cut my stepfather's hair wrong with the clippers just before his birthday. 'You did it to ruin my birthday!' Honestly, his short haircut was a welcome relief compared to that long grey hair, which mother had to grow back quickly as if he were the sex magnet of yesteryear.

My stepfather never hit me or abused me. Others did. He's not perfect, but I could undoubtedly have fared worse. I now know many who have fared worse. Some of them have been heaps of ashes for years. Others are inspired by how brightly they shine. Without exception, they are people. People need help. Only some don't have enough money to buy brushes. Others are blown away by legal jargon. I try to help these fellow sufferers as chairman of an interest group. My talents thus get a concrete application. A purpose. An action. It's not rest, it's activism. Much-needed activism.

I have bought a professional singing microphone. In my second year of pop-jazz at the singing academy, I'm learning to use my voice more and more correctly. My voice, which had disappeared on arrival at the psychiatric hospital. Whispering. Mumbling. Incomprehensible. I'm learning to tell my emotions more than to hold a tone. The singing teacher noticed I could produce something worth recording when I spread my wings. Something that both I and others will be amazed by. Sometimes, my voice is gone again. Then it comes back. It's mainly fun. I sing 'Summertime!' and I mean it. My new wheelchair was purchased with presentations in mind. The golden accents shine as brightly as I do.

On and off that stage, my beautiful, shiny black Labrador is always beside me. This certified Hachiko assistance dog helps me daily with lifting my legs, using the refrigerator, handing me things, taking off my trousers and jacket, opening and closing doors, and providing my phone if needed. He is the sweetest dog in the world. I cuddle him as often as possible.

I'm glad I waited until long after my admission to get this assistance dog, even though so many in my circle of acquaintances already had one. I didn't need one. I could do everything because I didn't have a disability. It's just a costly bicycle. And the same alcohol problem as my father. That's how my mother had raised me. This part of my past, and that's what it is now, is in the display cabinet. The figures I created are displayed at home as triumph pieces.

Today, I understand that the whirlwind was very often driven by the pain I experienced in my mother's long-standing refusal to acknowledge my emerging childhood traumas. The lack of a warm childhood cannot be adequately addressed in the clinical process of mental recovery. My therapist never cuddles me, either. Being open to cuddles is also challenging when the person before you pre-emptively bares their claws. Even though I choose to enter her open door again and again. The gap within myself is still very present. My ego is fragile. It still overwhelms me so often that my therapist has to remind me that I have to do it for myself. That the rest and their opinion of me can go to hell. Then I smile.

I make friends with almost everyone I meet. I can be proud of myself, love, and show what I am worth. From ashes, I can rise again and again. I have two children, ambitions, creations, opinions, relationships and a pause button to stop sending hate mail. I tell my children I love them and sleep in my wife's arms every night. Without exposing them to the self-harm with which I screamed out my helplessness. Although that whirlwind will never completely stop, the phoenix in me has taken full flight.

24 M.M.

Fortunately, I never experienced any neglect or abuse in any way whatsoever. My problems stem precisely from the fact that I received love and affection from my parents. But deep down, it gnaws at me, and I can't help but blame them for my unhappy childhood and hold them responsible for my unprocessed trauma. Unconsciously and unintentionally, they caused my overly sensitive daughter a great deal of suffering and never considered the consequences. They are wired differently to me, and they don't understand why I'm struggling, why I am the way I am, why I feel so abandoned and lonely.

I am from a South American country and moved here permanently around the age of nine to live with my mother and her husband. My mother left for here thirty-five years ago, following her love. There was no goodbye; I wasn't told I would miss her. My mother was gone, and I stayed behind with my father. In my memory, he did his best. He was solely responsible for my upbringing; there was no family nearby. It was just the two of us, which was good for me. I adored that man; he was the only person in my life. After all, my mother had abandoned me.

My parents rebuilt their lives with people I didn't know, one of whom I didn't even know existed. But they were there. My father remarried a colleague I'd never met. This woman moved in with us. Meanwhile, I longed for a mother figure in my life. I missed my mother terribly, but I had no one to fill that void. This woman couldn't and wouldn't, and her family even less so. I was ignored and, lest I forget, frequently told that I was a nuisance child who was in the way. My father also felt the need to have girlfriends, and I became the victim of his escapades. Those women took it out on me. For them, it was logical. You hurt our daughter, we hurt you, full stop!

Two years later, my mother returned to my life and took me to Belgium. I could live without my father, but not my mother; I knew that for sure. My suffering was over, and finally, I went on to happiness and an everyday life. Little did I know that I had, so to speak, died for my father then. It wasn't until ten years later that I saw him again, a stranger, disappointed to see a young woman and not his little nine-year-old daughter whom he'd lost.

My happiness and reunion with my mother were short-lived. Once in Belgium, I was dumped with my Belgian grandparents because my mother, due to her work, couldn't care for me. You're in a foreign country; you don't understand anything they're saying; the houses, the weather, and everything is different. I was lonely and alone. Again, I ended up in a family I didn't fit into, where I wasn't wanted. At least now, I had a name: the foreigner.

I was sent to boarding school when I became unmanageable for my mother. From the fourth year of primary school until the fifth year of secondary school, I learned to stand on my own two feet, take care of myself and stand up for myself. My childhood, like everyone else's, had its ups and downs. I was never thrilled but never unhappy, either.

When I first became a mother, everything slowly started to seep in. I would never let my child go through that, would I? Abandon him and entrust his care to someone else? Did my parents ever feel what I felt for my child? How can you abandon and leave your child? Was I ever truly loved?

When my psychiatrist sent his proposal to share the course of my illness and recovery, I didn't hesitate. If, through this, we can reach even just one person and encourage them to help themselves and believe in themselves, then I consider myself very fortunate. Unfortunately, there's still a huge taboo surrounding psychiatry and the people who are affected by it. We are put into boxes, let's say the 'normal' and the 'less normal'. Words like 'weak' and 'exaggerated' are often used. It's a shame because that's not how it is, not at all. Perception, a personal feeling, a personal experience. Yet I think the majority of fellow travellers will share this opinion.

It wouldn't happen to me again; I would feel it; I knew better; I'd been through it … until I couldn't take it anymore, and I fell apart in little pieces. I saw it coming, I felt it wasn't okay, but nobody listened. The GP dismissed me with new pills and told me I was 'highly sensitive'. No further explanation, no referral to a specialist, nothing.

Everything came together for me. My youngest son experienced depression, and I wasn't allowed to help him. My shaky relationship ended, and this was the proverbial straw that broke the camel's back. Suddenly, I was there, alone, written off, burnt out, mentally exhausted, sad and broken. I had fallen into a pit, a dark pit without a bottom. No matter how hard I tried to hold on to avoid sinking deeper, it didn't work. And above my head, the lid was closing more and more. In my head, it was chaos; my life was chaos. I saw myself lying there, broken into thousands of pieces, not knowing which piece to pick up first to begin rebuilding. Nothing made sense anymore; I was burnt out, I didn't care anymore. Fortunately, I didn't know what tsunami of pain and sorrow was about to hit me. Fortunately, I did realise that I needed help and sought it out. I was admitted to a PWGH ward. My stay there lasted eight weeks. Afterwards, I completed almost the entire process in a clinical psychotherapeutic ward of a PH (psychiatric hospital).

In the PWGH ward, I spoke with the psychologist, the psychiatrist and the nursing staff. Each was a strong support pillar guiding me through my world and inner turmoil. This was hell for me; I had the impression of having cried for eight weeks. It didn't stop. Soon, the conclusion was reached: I had a separation depression. Childhood traumas surfaced; my past caught up with me; I was presented with the bill. I never realised the impact of my not-so-happy and rosy childhood. Especially the sorrow I had suffered was still present somewhere. Deeply hidden and unprocessed grief. Towards the end of my stay, the carers and I realised that it wouldn't simply be resolved. The mess was too big to clear up in those eight weeks.

I tried to resume work, but the mountain was higher than I thought, and returning without the necessary support and peace of mind was impossible. The worst was the confrontation with my (then) ex-partner. We were and still are colleagues. For a week straight, I was brutally confronted with the reality of the separation, forced to see a reality I wasn't prepared for. I was ill, and he hadn't stopped to consider that. He had a new partner. It dawned on me that I missed him terribly and that he was one of the reasons I was giving up on my recovery.

In both the PWGH ward and the PH, the first week is a transitional, resting, and discovery phase. You don't yet participate in the activities; you need to acclimatise; you can rest your mind a bit. For me, it was quite the opposite; I found it very difficult, and it only made me more depressed. You have ample time to think, and I felt lost. On the other hand, that week allows you to get to know most of the people supporting you. You get the necessary explanations from everyone; you get the chance to tell your story; you are listened to. That's nice. Everything is interconnected; there's a reason for everything you do, and you learn more about your problem, especially yourself.

Contact with my fellow patients went smoothly, and I was immediately accepted into the group. It's unbelievable how quickly you bond with each other. You are supported in everything and feel you are not alone. At the same time, it is also challenging. Everyone has a heavy backpack, everyone has their problems, and everyone has their way of going through life. Precisely because you do almost everything together, you are also obliged to listen to the suffering of others. It is very intense to wrestle with yourself and to channel the other. Everything affects you enormously and strikes you. Some situations are harrowing, bordering on inhuman. All your energy is sucked away. It was intense, and I quickly tended to feel guilty. Yes, I was guilty. My problems seemed so much less significant compared to theirs because I wasn't strong enough. In my head, I had no reason to be there and was taking the place of someone who needed it more. These thoughts prevented me from entirely giving myself and exposing myself to everything. Not all the jars were opened, and I blocked a lot out. I only realised that after my admission in the last few months.

The approach in clinical psychotherapy is entirely different from that in the PWGH ward – a world of difference. Indeed, for people like me, where it's all much deeper hidden, everything there is based on talking, talking and more talking. I didn't believe in it; it made little sense; it wouldn't get me any further. Well, talking does help.

A simple drawing, song, or smell gets you thinking and talking. You are catapulted to your inner feelings, happiness and sadness, to a specific period, a good or a less good one. It's not easy, it's confronting, it's painful, it's revealing, it's everything. You touch one of your festering sores. From everyone – the psychiatrist, the psychologist, your internal supervisor – you get the necessary tools and support to start picking at these sores. It's up to you to do or postpone it because it will eventually come to the surface, tap you meanly on the shoulder, and show you clearly that it's there. Whether you like it or not. In my case, it took forty years. There was no place left to hide; everything was packed. Nobody shows you exactly how to do it; nobody takes over your thoughts to make it easier. It's your fight to the end. Fortunately, I had and still have, to this day, the reassurance and security of a large safety net.

Everyone who knows me well will agree that I like to laugh, try to stay positive and support someone through thick and thin, and I dare say it: I have a heart of gold. If necessary, I will step up for someone and not hesitate to make a fuss. I wear my heart on my sleeve, and if I genuinely love you, it's forever and unconditionally. I'm accused of being an incorrigible chatterbox with a good dose of self-confidence. Appearances can be deceiving, believe me. There's a dark side to me, a side I don't like to encounter or show. This makes me vulnerable, lonely and sad, without reason, without warning. This rears its head and knocks me flat. Everything I've rebuilt is swept away until I find the courage to rebuild again.

My admission lasted three months, and I didn't complete the entire process. I had dug enough into my past, and it wasn't working financially either. My benefits had become too low to be able to pay for everything at home; after all, I was alone again. Against the wishes of my supervisor and the psychiatrist, I stopped and picked up the threads again.

It wasn't easy to get used to the outside world again. I hadn't yet severed the umbilical cord with the hospital. I missed the safe feeling, an environment where I could be myself without prejudice. But the clinic wasn't my home, nor was it my life. From then on, the 'again' period started. Again, I had to let go without knowing how. Again, I felt lonely in my struggle, falling and getting up, again long conversations with the psychologist, again everything. Life has challenged me a lot; it has cost me much effort not to give up.

Five years later, I am still building and learning to accept and love myself. I am still under the care of a psychiatrist. When things get tough again, I automatically talk to a psychologist. When the fear is there again, I know it will also pass. I'm getting better at being my old self again, even though I realise I'll never fully be that person again. My life is divided into two chapters: before and after my admission. I often refer to my illness as 'the beast'. It's inside me, and sometimes it rages through my body. Who knows if my struggle will ever end? It might, we'll see, I don't want to know.

Today, five years later, I try to find happiness in small things. The better and happier periods are predominant. Now that I know myself, I have more control and try to keep it that way. I know it doesn't always work, but that's how it works for me. We keep it that way. My glass is half full again; I would never have dared to dream that. Sometimes, dreams do come true.

25 M.V.

I was born the fourth child, unwanted (I heard that almost every day); I felt worthless and like a burden. What happened in my life marked me; I was bullied at school because I had red hair and freckles, the Pippi Longstocking syndrome. At age ten, I changed from a mixed school to a girls' (and nuns') school, which, if possible, made me even less keen to go to school. At the age of thirteen, my favourite aunt died; I couldn't say goodbye or grieve. I had to follow a path that wasn't my choice at all. The Child Guidance Centre and my parents decided for me. At seventeen, I started working in a factory; I didn't want to go to school anymore but wanted to marry as soon as possible to get away from home. After a year, I moved to another factory, where a fire broke out at my machine. The questioning and accusations were very humiliating; I didn't even get support from my parents. In the early years of our marriage, we also had many setbacks: my husband had a serious accident, I had a miscarriage, another miscarriage after two children, financial problems, and my husband's long working hours made things extra difficult for me. My father's illness and death twenty-five years ago had a significant impact on me. Then, the health problems started, followed by mental health problems. This led to a breakdown a year later.

I had low self-esteem, felt like a burden and worthless, and had no more interest in my own family or life. I lost my zest for life, withdrew into myself, and wore a mask. I constantly had suicidal thoughts, couldn't bear anything anymore, felt short-changed, and was a bad mother because of my behaviour towards the children.

At the end of that year, I contacted my GP, who diagnosed depression and arranged for admission to a psychiatric ward (PWGH). At that time, depression and psychiatry were a huge taboo. During this admission, it was mainly medication that gave me a numb feeling. I felt like a zombie, and my weight increased, which became an additional problem. A year later, I attempted suicide very seriously. Only then was my depression seriously addressed. But in the wrong way for me. I had absolutely no expectations, only a death wish. After several suicide attempts and admissions to various psychiatric wards, I was admitted to a clinical psychotherapeutic ward of a psychiatric hospital. It's a clinic I didn't want to go to; it was known as the 'madhouse'. You never got out of there.

I heard my diagnosis from the assistant psychiatrist: dysthymic disorder, borderline personality disorder and dissociative identity disorder – that's what I still remember. A life sentence, I thought and felt for a long time. Also, something you can hide behind. I wanted to return to the old life as soon as possible. Something that happened quite quickly. After a month of full-time admission, I went to day therapy. This allowed me to spend time with the children during the summer holidays and leave the clinic as quickly as possible. Because of this, I only did what was necessary for the therapies to protect myself, something that largely succeeded, with occasional short periods of full admission. I was fully discharged in September of the following year and switched to outpatient therapy.

During this admission, I experienced psychotherapy as a necessity, a compulsion. I diligently followed all the prescribed and freely chosen therapies. The group sessions were challenging at first. I didn't like the group psychologist at all. I constantly annoyed myself with him, what he did or didn't do, how he spoke or remained silent. He couldn't do anything right in my eyes. When a childhood trauma (sexual abuse) surfaced, I was angry with him. However, that was necessary so I could work on it. In group therapy, I was more concerned with changing others than myself. It frustrated me that fellow patients didn't follow therapy so strictly. I found many therapies useless and time-filling.

Back home, I felt strong and sound and looked for and found a job. I wanted to contribute to the family and have something to do during the day. The fact that I took a low-paying job was a minor detail at the time. I continued outpatient therapy for a year. Due to a mishap, I cancelled all outpatient appointments; I thought I could manage on my own now.

I felt good; I didn't realise I was already running away, an old pattern, instead of tackling it. A year later, a total crash was more profound than ever before. Full admission again; I was utterly overwhelmed. I was entirely without expectations then; no one could help me. Those were difficult months; it became four-and-a-half years, alternating between full admission and day therapy, discharge and relapse. A period that I used to delve into, to see, to process and to change. The expectation was to function again as a wife, mother and housekeeper at home.

Psychotherapy became a help, a tool to get better, to get to know myself and to accept myself. I worked very intensively and experienced many difficult periods and confinement in the seclusion room to protect myself from myself in case of too much threat or after an attempt. I learned to recognise the signals in myself to ask for isolation myself. This safety allowed me to go deeper into the therapies. Today, I probably look at treatment very differently than I did then. I learned that everyone has their truth, how I see it and how someone else sees it. Another replaced the group psychologist; this didn't go smoothly; the previous one was suddenly better, but that changed quickly. This one had a very different approach, or so it felt. It took some getting used to, but I was already better at talking and maybe also at manipulating, which (in retrospect, I think) I did now and then. With this therapist, it started to click, and I could deeply understand our conversations. He also became my outpatient therapist after admission for many years. I diligently and meticulously followed all therapies. Only in the last admissions did I learn to neglect therapy. I learned to play truant, so to speak. The fear of being punished was gone.

According to your assigned group, I had a fixed programme in both admissions. You also had the choice of sessions in the forum for personality development. I was assigned to group C, which was unpleasant because it indicated your problem. At a certain point, the letters were replaced by a number. Group C became 4. C4 had something explosive for me (*M.K.*: in B., this stands for dismissal by the employer); it had a nasty connotation.

All therapies have helped me in one way or another. I only realised this later (for many). Psycho- or talk therapies have, in retrospect, helped a lot. Getting to know yourself through this and how you view, experience and perceive something. Both individual and group therapies. The practical therapies (such as the household programme at the time) helped to give the group a better understanding. We need more trust in each other to talk better and more freely. It also brought annoyance and discussion, which could be addressed with guidance.

Communication training was the most annoying therapy – unnecessary, just irritating. It consisted of a series that was repeated. I followed this many times. The repetition ingrained it, which was a great help after psychiatry. I still consciously use it every day. In the second admission, this was dropped, and only then did I notice how good this was.

The living activities were a pleasant affair where you learned to respect each other, where you learned to accept defeat in the game, and where I took up needlework again. It taught me to get back into the mother role and care for my children. I experienced occupational therapy as 'annoying therapy'. I had difficulty getting along with the therapist. I experienced it as having to follow the rules, although I eventually achieved beautiful things there.

Expressive therapy helped me clearly express what was going on inside me through visual expression. It did make me dislike making collages. Our group was chosen as a test group for dance therapy. What resistance we offered! Showing your expression through dance, however closed or open you are. The resistance gradually disappeared, and it was something to look forward to later – relaxing movement and daring to be more open in a safe environment.

The individual supervisor was my support and confidante during my various admissions. I had many supervisor changes and had difficulty with that. But they were all, in their way, excellent help for me during many arduous periods.

To complete this, I will also tell you about the activities chosen for personality development in the forum. 'Eye-opener' was an enriching therapy for me. I followed this for a very long time. I had a good click with the two therapists there. It was an in-depth therapy, yet relaxing and fun. Sometimes, it is very intense but very clarifying and problem-solving. Furthermore, I followed various choices, including shiatsu massage and reflexology. Later, I even followed a reflexology course. This has become my passion and my job!

At the time, there were many therapies that I didn't find helpful. Later, I realised how much it all had worked. What helped less were the weekly general meetings and the process guidance. What I also didn't experience as help were the changes that took place a few times. Change in group name, change of group supervision, different psychologist (that was actually for the better), changing assistants, changes in nursing and therapies.

My psychotherapeutic process, therefore, took a very long time. This process never stops. I now describe it as personal growth and development. After admission came outpatient therapy. Weekly with the psychologist and monthly with the psychiatrist. The latter became less frequent and stopped four years ago. After years, I changed psychologists.

It was a long, difficult road because I resisted it for the first few years. Also, because my problems were quite significant, I still had a complicated relationship with my mother and sister. The environment also slows down a process because they don't accept your change. Because of this, people have disappeared from my life, and my relationship with them has changed. Because in the first admission, I only wanted to become the old me, I relapsed into old habits and old behaviour, which caused problems again. My husband remained by my side; we have grown together in our relationship and gone through it together. Fortunately, I got the time to work on myself and become who I am today. It is something that I take with me in my life, use, and constantly improves me.

Due to the long and numerous admissions, the transition back home was difficult. It felt unsafe and uncertain. The house had become the clinic for me. As if I had become unwelcome at home, my place was gone. I had to regain that; with the proper support, I was helped through this. At this point, I was still a very dependent woman. Making my own decisions was already a bit better; I had also gained many insights, but there was still a long way to go.

I now had interests that I wanted to develop by following training; reflexology became my passion. The enjoyment and satisfaction I found in it led to the decision to make it my profession. To do this, I needed additional training: a massage therapist. Now, I could start my own business at my own pace, and with the hours, I could manage it without losing my replacement income. I could create my own job with the psychiatrist's and my family's support. I have learned to stand up for myself and to seize and create opportunities.

Everything that has happened, all the treatments, and all the people I have come into contact with have made me who I am today. It has given me a lot of self-knowledge and knowledge of how to interact with others and stand in life. I am very grateful for this, which has given me enormous strength and self-confidence.

My evolution was slow but increasingly accelerated. It was a complex, arduous process, with highs and enormous lows, extremes. I think I was one of the most 'difficult' patients. There came stability and regularity; I became more substantial and more self-confident. A setback no longer completely knocked me down, and I knew where I could go, which was enormous support. My own business gave me prospects, which made me better and better. I have undergone tremendous growth. Something I am proud of. My diagnosis was significant and burdensome, a stigma. Today, I am an example of how you can erase that stigma. If you are willing to change, you can be who you want to be. A bad day is not bad; it is a day to reflect and consider what is happening.

I live today; I live in the now. If a problem arises, I tackle it. A problem disappears when the solution appears. I am a satisfied person and happy with what I have today. My future is to continue growing, discovering, and undertaking, and as a wife, mother and grandmother, enjoying many moments of life. Further developing my business, organising retreats, working with groups or individually. Supporting people to become aware and create their happiness. Good self-care, facing the future with an open mind, grateful for what is. My growth is what I am today and who I can become tomorrow.

26 N.A.

Psychotherapy wasn't something I consciously chose; I somewhat stumbled into it. Seeking urgent help for my low mood, anxiety, resulting sleep problems and yet another low point in my life, I ended up seeing a psychiatrist through a friend. I'd previously seen psychologists who listened attentively, but the conversations lacked depth, remaining superficial. There were also long gaps between sessions. And as for medication, the psychologist wasn't qualified to prescribe appropriate support. The intake with the psychiatrist was different to what I was used to – more thorough. My family tree was drawn up and explored. What I found positive and more personal was that the people who played a role in my life were given names, not numbers or figures.

During the initial sessions, I mainly outlined my current situation: relationship problems, low self-esteem and a growing susceptibility to addictions – alcohol, nicotine and sleeping pills. As the sessions progressed, we got to the root of the problem: my childhood, adolescence, relationship with my parents and the loss of a loved one. I didn't realise these were the roots of my apparent abandonment issues.

My childhood and teenage years weren't exactly the happiest. My father, a self-employed house painter, was more absent than present. My mother gave my brother and me the impression that we were unwanted, using words like: 'You two are the nails in my coffin.' We were very young when she sent us out to work, though she always found us weekend and holiday jobs – as long as we stayed out of her way. I left home immediately, settling with my partner at eighteen. He was my rock for thirteen years. He saw my talent, gave me confidence, and enabled me to develop and do things I was good at. He fell madly in love with my best friend in his final year. He was in his late twenties when he died in a car accident.

That's when I started taking antidepressants and sleeping pills for support. We had a large circle of friends, and I received good support in the years following his death. However, I still missed the affection and warmth of someone close to me. That's how I ended up with the man who is my daughter's father. I was unexpectedly pregnant after six weeks. Becoming a mother – a word with a negative connotation for me.

He was a good father to the children but couldn't fill the void of the love I'd missed from my mother. I didn't realise at the time that no one could. A married man came into my life when my need for affection peaked. He understood my frustration and pain; we were in the same boat. He regretted his marriage vows. I felt sorry for him because he was tied down, and I felt much less in my current relationship.

My partner had never proposed. Deep down, I was saddened and sometimes angry. For a long time, I felt I was good enough to be the mother of his children, but nothing more. I would never be his wife. The married man and I began a secret relationship. We clicked. After a few months, I wanted to reveal our secret, but he didn't. His wife hadn't done anything wrong, and he didn't want to hurt her. He wanted to continue the lies; I didn't. My trust in him rapidly diminished when I learned I was just the latest in a long line of mistresses. Because I didn't want to deny myself affection, the relationship only ended after over three years, after I informed his wife. She covered the whole thing up.

That experience left me feeling like I'd lost again. I felt abandoned, or rather, betrayed and lied to. Similarly, my relationship with the father of my children ended after twenty years. My search for love and affection continued. I clung to anyone I thought could fill the void. Friends and some female friends felt suffocated by my behaviour. A couple of men even said I was 'clawing at their skin', resulting in people turning their backs on me, leaving me deeply hurt.

At that point, I was devastated. I spiralled downwards, feeling intensely guilty about having brought two children into the world whom I couldn't properly care for – for whom, like my mother, I was emotionally unavailable. Fortunately, the psychotherapy had already started. I got to know myself better. Gradually, it became clear how I kept ending up in this vicious cycle. I attracted the wrong men in my quest for validation, love and affection. The basic needs, once met by my deceased partner and previously by my late grandmother, who lived with us during my childhood, disappeared with their deaths. This significant loss plagued my life. My mother never put me on her lap, sending me to boarding school instead. Perhaps she couldn't show love to her children because she had missed it, which was unknown to her.

The therapy sessions were challenging, sometimes painful, at first, but they were weekly, which reassured me. Salvation was never far away. The therapist never offered unsolicited advice or judgement. They only provided guidance if I explicitly asked for it. Instead, they might make a witty reference to a film or book to illustrate or clarify situations. Occasionally, a proverb or saying would be quoted, which I could then work with. If I lingered too long on current events, the therapist would gently point out that while current events were important, we should focus on the matter at hand.

After each session, I had food for thought and the feeling that a weight had been lifted. The sessions were beneficial and provided insight, encouraging self-reflection. It felt like I could leave my sadness behind – a shared sorrow is half a sorrow, as they say. My burden felt lighter and lighter. Now, I barely carry it at all. Through psychotherapy, I can contribute more to others in their search for peace or when they are stuck in life. I'd already been a listening ear for my clients in my profession. My feedback helps them, given that they request it. I'm grateful I was able to have psychotherapy, though unfortunately, the cost (mainly with psychologists) is a barrier for some. Good therapists are often busy, and finding one can be difficult, especially in crises. I navigate life more calmly now, thanks to the insight I've gained into myself and others.

27 N.S.

My life can be read as a string of meaningless sacrifices and absurd commands. Experience taught me that everything life offers is vain and unreliable. My parents had a silly, unscrupulous way of thinking and acting. I wanted to escape this futility. But there is no escape. You know, and you don't know. My brother and I were very introverted. We did not need to express ourselves or talk. We had learned to accept everything, to be polite and, above all, to remain silent. The art was to be as unobtrusive as possible. The keys to my youth are worthless. None of them fit the gates of success. My parents made us weak, but they claimed to have 'improved' us.

I have a history of physical, sexual and emotional abuse and neglect – the abuses I experienced as a child within the family. As a child, I had been disturbed in my contact with sexuality. Incest. My sense of safety had been impaired. I also had a crippling fear of failure. I was tuned in to fear, danger, risk and suspicion. The suffering was not just emotional damage; I also had problems with my memory, learning and attention.

My earliest memories are of anxiously wondering what would happen next. There were permanent tensions in our home. You can't say it as a child, but you're 'in' it. The impression of that time at home was that I had no ground under my feet, no basis to build on. Everything revolved around power. The greater ruling over the smaller, the stronger over the weaker, the man over the woman. The worst in that period was the feeling that I had to endure, not show that I couldn't cope anymore. To escape was to perish. I had to drag myself through a shallow river full of mud. Sometimes, I felt I had to bear the responsibility for the entire family. Anything was possible in our home, but nothing was to be understood. There were no norms and values. My childhood was marked by their attempts to increase their power.

My brother and I lived in poverty at home, but it was not visible. The food was in a separate garage that only my father could access. He liked to have control over us. My brother and I suffered much hunger. To the outside world, we were the rich kids for many. To survive, I had to create my world. Turn off my feelings and put my thoughts on autopilot. This worked for quite some time.

Ten years ago, I ended up in 'psychiatry' in September. My husband pointed out that I was quickly irritated and warned me about my behaviour. I also had a serious alcohol problem. Not that I drank in a daze. I wanted to feel normal. I dragged my environment into my chaos and my issues. I forced my environment into my disturbed way of functioning. I was constantly in a state of anxiety, increased irritability, insomnia and nightmares, and I was hyperalert. My nightmares completely threw me off. I dreamed of a volcanic eruption, and I had no more ground. There was only lava. Every day again. Enough to drive you crazy. From others, I've heard that I crossed the street on foot without looking, and other cars had to avoid me. I can't remember anything about it. I had to fight the urge to commit suicide. I had outright suicidal tendencies. My GP noticed that I had lost much weight in a very short time. I said I was a bit stressed but couldn't express what was happening in my head. She said she wanted to see me weekly. Emotionally, I completely closed off, as if I was completely numb. Paralysed. I just stared ahead. I felt 'detached' from time, as if it wasn't there. Through my GP, I was then admitted twice for two months in a PWGH.

I had flashbacks and intrusive thoughts. I was in a constant state of excitement. It was precisely stored energy stuck in my body, not only in my body but also in my head. I started to become very aggressive. I fought out of blind rage as if I was in a trance. I was no longer in control of myself. The reactions were more instinctive than well considered, more unconscious than conscious. For my safety and that of the other patients, I was sometimes sent to the isolation cell, usually bound for the first hours. It was the only place where I felt safer. Not that there weren't any more fears. The flashbacks were there, but there were no new triggers and fewer external stimuli. Sometimes, I asked the psychiatrist if I could go to the isolation cell for a few hours. I felt powerless and desperate. I fled into my imagination. The conversations with the psychologist were difficult. I kept the lid on my memory firmly closed because I thought that was better. In consultation with the team, long-term assistance in a specialised psychiatric facility was proposed. It was already a whole 'transformation' for me to know what I had a name for: complex PTSD (post-traumatic stress disorder). My treatment lasted a total of five years during my stay.

Through my flashbacks, I was overwhelmed by blind rage. I had tried to banish the anger from my heart, but the loudest language was that of violence. An uncomfortable tension had nestled in my head, and a predator was waiting for a chance to break out in my ribcage. I felt overwhelmed and lost. I felt like a phoenix being consumed by its fire. Every week, I have a weekly schedule with fixed therapeutic activities divided into verbal and non-verbal activities. The fixed therapies included weekend discussion, music, expression, process (course of your treatment), sport, ergo, individual psycho, group psycho, conversation with my PN (personal nurse), psycho-education and weekend evaluation. There were modules such as mentalisation, dialectical behavioural therapy and the wellness recovery action plan (WRAP). There was also a choice of around 80 forum activities: trauma and recovery; I was a CPMP child, dreams, philosophical workshop, resilience, sports, mindfulness, etc. Expression had the most profound impact. So deep that I sometimes only had sensory impressions of trauma and no conscious ones. The interesting thing about expression is that you can use images from prints to describe the depth of trauma. With words, it was much more difficult. Through the pictures, more and more memories came back. What struck me was that with each image, the impact of the first traumatic event was reinforced and automatically added to it. After the expression, I always felt excited, to the extent that I forgot reality. I fled into my imagination. The drives were suddenly there. This often manifested itself in aggression towards materials. It wasn't easy to translate thoughts and feelings into meaningful words. It was also challenging to symbolise my experiences, so they did not gain meaning.

I began to have an internal conflict between intrusiveness and avoidance. I wanted to forget, suppress, deny and minimise. With the psychotherapist, I slowly began to talk about fragments from the past. I began to realise that I could take more by talking about it. The anger was still there, but it was no longer blind rage. I learned better to connect my feelings to my thoughts and memories. I learned to pause and question my thoughts, feelings and memories. Certain elements were explored in depth. I also learned to reflect on what was emotionally happening to me. I had an individual session with the psychologist every week and a group session twice a week. The advantage of an individual session is that I could go deeper into my problems. I often wondered what she would read in my words. Whether she would understand me? Would I be condemned for it? I also asked if she would believe me. So much had happened.

Often, unwanted childhood memories colonised my retina. Sometimes, normal feelings, thinking and speaking became too real for me. Before and after the sessions, I had to masturbate compulsively. It was also excruciating to realise how my parents were. I then began to reverse the roles and say that I was terrible. What also shocked me was that my memory was not infallible. My brother had a diary, and I concluded that certain elements did not match my brother's elements. Memory is not a film that records something and can later be rewound and watched again. It is more malleable, manipulable and suggestible when given, just like the imagination. We look at it how we want it to be, not how it is. It's like the sun. Even though we know the sun doesn't revolve around the Earth, we still imagine it that way and say: the sun rises and sets.

In group psychotherapy, I was in a group where the most essential part of the recovery was that there was a sense of safety. 'What is said within these four walls stays within those walls' was a powerful rule. An essential part of the group process was sharing traumatic events and their meaning with the group. The psychologist re-exposes you to the memory of the events to desensitise you to them. It's about making sense of something incomprehensible. The psychologist paid attention to the impact of the trauma on someone's attitude towards safety and danger, trust and self-image. I did my best to 'reason' social behaviour and people and to analyse them intellectually. At first, I felt like a spectator in the back row on the sidelines. The idea was to free associate. To learn to speak without a filter. The initiative was expected on a social and communicative level. That was a big challenge for me because I was not only afraid of being overwhelmed by feelings, but I was also highly socially anxious.

I was also afraid to confess my actions and desires because then I would expose myself to the judgement of others. At first, I found it pointless to express everything you think. You create opinions that would have been better never born. Rows that get out of hand, one word provokes another; someone gets aggressive, and why? There's nothing to gain. I had regular run-ins with other patients. I have learned a lot about human behaviour and reactions. After half a year, I started talking, albeit sparingly, but I had started. But it wasn't simple. In the beginning, my language was mainly egocentric. Certainly not to interact. A storm of emotions came up – shame, guilt, fear and anger. Also, there are palpitations, sweating and the feeling of losing self-control. I was always asking myself questions, like why a particular person, in a specific context, had those thoughts. Yet, it doesn't provide much clarity. Every person is different. You have to look at it individually. The thoughts of a thinker are always a kind of autobiography, albeit an unwitting one. Through speaking, thoughts can gradually emerge.

From the caregivers, I found it essential that they want to get to know you. Not just hear, but listen. I also liked calm and assertive therapists. I also found the care necessary. Every patient also had an individual supervisor. Mutual trust was a must, I thought. It creates a bond. As a caregiver, being credible is essential; otherwise, everything will fail from the start. By plausible, I mean being your true self. I wouldn't come to a trusting relationship if this were constantly hidden. I learned a lot during my psychiatric hospitalisation.

After my psychiatric discharge, I am in outpatient therapy with the same psychiatrist. Rationally, I thought a lot had been processed and was behind me until I got stuck on specific topics that I still relived. But even more intense than before. By talking about it more and more, reliving it, all the elements come back to life. I also often had nervous, unpleasant sensations in my body. Ultimately, I have learned that bodily sensation is a significant source of information. How I am evolving now, I can best compare to the renovations of my house. There were many defects, so a lot had to be demolished again to be rebuilt. In psychiatry, I could still carefully hide many signals. In outpatient therapy, this is much less possible. It is no longer possible for me to suppress my feelings. Sometimes, everything floods in, and then I feel caught and attacked. The therapy is much more intensive. The problems can be better studied. The frequency of the treatment is also higher. Now it's twice a week. What is necessary to get to know someone thoroughly? The more intensive it becomes, the faster you get to the point. It's not easy for me because I'm afraid of losing control. My emotions then become very intense. You don't want to feel hurtful, shameful or disgusting feelings. But you have no other choice. Every morning holds a threat: flashbacks, fears, powerlessness, hopelessness. You only live out of obligations, out of habits, but without conviction. It became more and more clear to me how, for years, I have been suppressing my feelings and what weird and fatal reaction patterns have emerged in the area of human relationships as a result. My psychiatrist tries to provide a thoughtful insight into the complex whole.

More and more, I see my psychiatrist as a father figure. Someone I look up to. Someone who gives me the motivation to learn and keep going. Someone I trust.

Someone who sets boundaries is professional and can think outside the box. In my first year in psychiatry, I felt very ill at ease with the psychiatrist. I felt vulnerable, not at all protected. I came from a primitive environment. There were no norms and values. I didn't detect any similarities. I also had little academic knowledge. I gradually realised that he did not judge me. He assumed you could still acquire that knowledge if you had little knowledge. It was crucial to me that there was understanding at that moment, as I was, even though change had to come. I focus less on previous behaviours because I am more aware of my limits and barriers. Now, I pay more attention to my feelings and signals from within me. The path to be travelled is difficult. It is a path of toiling and crying, of no longer being able to, of not sleeping, of anger, of fighting, of holding on and letting go. My acting, doing and deciding were based primarily on my emotions. Now, I look at life more scientifically – rationally. I see therapy as a signpost that enables me to handle, question and live myself more intensely and qualitatively. Ultimately, I believe in gradual progress. It is necessary to give yourself the time. You have to experience and feel what you have suppressed. I notice this as my body begins to speak. It doesn't use tricks to get through. Dreams are also significant in knowing what's going on inside you. After much toil and work, many fundamental things have already been restored. My perception as a person has expanded. I am more aware of myself. Yet, there are still blocks that I have to continue working on in therapy.

28 P.D.M.

I started clinical psychotherapy because of a severe depression that had been dragging on for years and was triggered again by the death of my father. I also had persistent anorexia nervosa. Furthermore, I struggled with a general feeling of complete lethargy and weariness of life. Forming relationships was also complicated. I lived at home with my parents, and we formed a trinity that wasn't okay for anyone. I wanted to break free and go my own way, but I had no idea how.

Before that, I had been in outpatient treatment with various psychologists for a long time. That didn't prevent me from making a severe suicide attempt that resulted in a coma. After that, I had a very long residential treatment. This admission, however, ended again with a serious suicide attempt that almost resulted in blindness. I knew deep down that it couldn't go on like this (not only for myself but also for those around me). My friends and relatives were also afraid that I would attempt suicide again, and some thought it would end in suicide.

A certain calmness came over me at the moment I let myself be admitted. I was freed from the world, and others were now taking over for me. It did feel like a liberation. I could finally sleep properly for the first time in a long time. I didn't expect much. I had already given myself up somewhat. I had already accepted the possibility of spending the rest of my days in an institution; strangely, I was at peace with that. The world was too complex a place for me. I had also built up an overly idealistic image of the world. I couldn't cope with the real world. Incidentally, this is still difficult to this day.

It was challenging for me to express my feelings in words at the time. I was unable to speak honestly. First and foremost, allowing myself to feel my feelings was very difficult. Perhaps those feelings would be too great, too violent? In addition, there was little connection with my body. More than anything, I wanted to 'disappear' from the world. My anorexia was a kind of alternative suicide. It was also a way to be 'small', literally to take up almost no space; I didn't want to grow. I continued to struggle with the question of whether you should live simply because you were born. This question never left me. I also always read many pessimistic and/or melancholic writers such as Cioran, Arendt, Bataille, Kierkegaard, Schopenhauer, Musil and many great (melancholic) Russians. I also read much poetry.

I resisted the therapy with all my might, but there was a clear need for help. I wasn't always aware of this, but still … It took a long time before I let the therapists in. I found the actual 'speaking' difficult, even though I had already sought help, both outpatient and residential, for quite some time.

I found the psychotherapy threatening. Expressing feelings in a group was difficult, especially since I had minimal contact with my feelings. Because of my anorexia nervosa, I had also cut myself off from my feelings. I weighed barely forty kilograms and looked like someone who had just come from Buchenwald (concentration camp), and my body, therefore, first and foremost, had to ensure its physical survival. Much energy went into simply maintaining my body, so there was very little room left for proper therapy.

I both wanted and didn't want to 'cooperate' and made things difficult for myself and the therapist. Did I want to be helped, to 'get better'? A power struggle arose between me and the psychiatrist. Thanks to his angelic patience, I can now put these reflections on paper. Everything is repeated in a therapeutic process. The ward, acting as a mother, and the psychiatrist acting as a father (for me, anyway), meant that the struggle that must have been there in my early childhood between and within this trinity erupted again with full force.

I found the therapeutic process very difficult. At some moments there was cooperation, and I may even have behaved docilely; at other times, there was rebellion, and I refused all cooperation. At those times, I boycotted myself and the therapist, often leading to impasses between us. How frequently must the psychiatrist have considered referring me to a chronic ward because I couldn't or wouldn't be helped?

It took a long time before any therapeutic process (in the group) could take place. In the meantime, I sometimes intervened, but starting to talk about myself seemed difficult. Did I not want to, couldn't I, or did I want to make it difficult for the therapist? It's a combination of the three. Working on myself meant I would have to detach myself from my mother and take responsibility for myself. That's precisely what I didn't want or couldn't do. I could take responsibility for someone else, but it was challenging.

I was sometimes afraid of the psychiatrist. He could be steadfast at times. I would then retreat into myself and completely 'block'. I still suffer from this. I also idealised the therapist and attributed great power to him. I may have sometimes expected him to utter a redeeming word at some point, solving all my problems. At the same time, I also fought with him. It wasn't easy. I wanted to cooperate, and at the same time, I did nothing but rebel. I had very ambivalent feelings towards the therapist. That duality and ambivalence have been playing a role throughout my life.

It's the same ambivalence that I undoubtedly always felt towards my father and my mother. Of course, that ambivalence was also present on their part, making things very difficult between us sometimes. There was always an alliance of two people against the other person. However, this alliance constantly changed, making it all very confusing for me.

The same ambivalence also occurred throughout my therapy towards nurses and therapists (and actually, how could it be otherwise, also towards myself). It undoubtedly caused a lot of misunderstandings and conflicts and created a bizarre phenomenon: I am terrified of disputes, but because of my way of being, I sometimes provoke conflicts. I can't seem to escape this, or perhaps I don't want to because I know it so well. Boundaries were also very fluid in the family I grew up in.

Undoubtedly, many different factors helped. I benefited a lot from the painting studio. Dance therapy (to restore my relationship with my body) also did me good. In addition, I was also lucky to have the opportunity to stay in the centre for a long time. Having time also helped. Speaking out about certain things – albeit after a long time – also helped immensely. Speaking out is already very good; the 'just keep talking' is still problematic. This speaking out wasn't easy, and I often had to recover from a psychotherapeutic session in which something was said and certain things became visible. Even when the gate to truth/awareness is wide open, there is sometimes an immense hesitation/fear to step over the threshold. The interaction with the other group members was certainly interesting and educational.

At a certain point, you act as a mirror for the other, and that difference, in turn, acts as a mirror for you. There were also conflicts in the group. I couldn't cope with that. I still can't cope with conflicts. I then block, become sad, and would rather disappear from the world. It's not the right way to act, but it's still my attitude.

The unwavering, non-judgemental presence of the nursing staff also helped a lot. These people's patience was incredible, and I can only be grateful. Even though I didn't always make it easy for them, I could always go to them. During my admission, I also read a lot. I have always found comfort in books and the words of (in my eyes) 'Great Men'. They are my last resort. When I am no longer able to read because I cannot concentrate, I know that things are not going too well with me. This is usually followed by a period in which I am somewhat lethargic and turn away from the world.

What indeed didn't help were my rebelliousness, lack of feeling, ambivalence, split personality and introverted character. Also, 'language' was completely absent in our family in early childhood. This resulted in little connection with my mother and minimal 'language' between my parents.

It all took so long because of too much resistance. There was too little interest in myself to get better. My persistent anorexia nervosa also made it take a long time. I was literally in survival mode. All the remaining energy that was still present in my emaciated body was primarily used to survive. There was simply no energy to work therapeutically. It took a long time because, at times, I didn't care anymore. Being admitted forever, I had made peace with that.

Why put more energy into something that might mean I wouldn't be admitted? The idea of returning to that oh-so-difficult real world for me was terrifying, so I didn't cooperate in a process that might make and hasten this return possible.

I was in full admission for a long time: almost a year-and-a-half or so. After that, there was a long period of day therapy. The day therapy was necessary because my anorexia hadn't disappeared yet and also especially to give structure to my days. The structure is something difficult for me. In my childhood, there had been little fundamental structure. Without day therapy, it was not inconceivable that I would, for example, walk around in my pyjamas until noon and that I would again end up in a kind of hopeless, lethargic existence. It helped me find a precarious balance between the world inside (the institution) and the world outside. That wasn't even the real world. It was the world as I knew it. After my long admission, I returned to live with my mother. It was probably not such a good idea, but for me, it was self-evident at that time.

After that, I went for outpatient treatment on Monday evenings (group therapy) for a long time. I was admitted residentially twice in the following years – each time for a shorter period. During my second admission, the psychiatrist 'forced' me to look for a house or apartment. I had to go and live alone. My anorexia had disappeared by my last admission.

In the meantime, I had travelled a lot, and during one of these trips, I started eating deliciously again, and it could even be a bit more. I even started to enjoy life. Since then, I occasionally visit my psychiatrist (from back then). I see a psychotherapist almost weekly and have done so for many years. I have never been without therapy since my admission.

In the meantime, I am free of my anorexia nervosa. I can sleep better. There are still periods when I suffer from insomnia, especially when it's too busy in my head. Then those feelings from 'back' come back: sadness, grief, anger ... Unfortunately, I am still not able to express that anger verbally. I still turn the anger against myself in the form of depressive feelings. I also struggle to concentrate and catch myself being a bit 'absent' in the world. I then retreat into myself again and shut myself off. I am then doing myself a disservice. My self-esteem should undoubtedly be a bit higher after all that therapy.

My suicidal thoughts have more or less subsided. There are still periods when I wouldn't necessarily consider death an unwelcome guest, but still ...

My inner restlessness has decreased (there are still periods when I am restless and can't sleep well). I am less lethargic, but I catch myself having such a period now and then. I now have an adorable wife who loves and cares for me. I try to take good care of her in my way, too. I more or less succeed in building up and maintaining a specific structure. I have been working part-time for ten years now. Before my admission, I had hardly ever worked.

I look back on my process with mixed feelings. Was it all worth it? I honestly don't know sometimes. Life remains difficult for me. However, I am grateful that, through all that therapy, I have my lovely wife, whom I would never have met otherwise. She teaches me daily that unconditional love exists and cares for me. She also lets me be myself, even if that is sometimes 'a somewhat melancholic' person. I still don't feel strong enough, and I remain fragile. Too little self! It's a shaky building with too little foundation. A strong storm, and I'll be knocked over.

I want to work for a few more years and study philosophy. I have always enjoyed having my head in books and still consider them a refuge. When the world is too 'scary' for me, they catch me. Sad? Maybe, but that's just the way it is. I hope to stop going to psychotherapists one day. I sometimes have to let go of things, but I still can't do that well enough. Not everything can be solved; not all questions can be answered. I also enjoy travelling and would like to do it often. Above all, I hope the love between me and my wife will continue to last. Without her, I think I am lost again. That's too bad, but I fear that would be the case. I don't know whether I would still have the courage to start again.

While writing this story, I thought of the verses of Paul Verlaine: *C'est bien la pire peine/De ne savoir pourquoi/Sans amour et sans haine/Mon coeur a tant de peine!* (It's the worst pain/Not to know why/Without love or hate/My heart is so sad!) Meanwhile, I better understand why it sometimes rains heavily and storms in my heart.

29 P.S.

'A boy who has experienced emotional neglect feels the need to prove himself in every possible way. He manifests himself and cries out for the attention he didn't receive.' This accurately describes my background, complemented by an inferiority complex ... During my artistic studies and active career, I gave one hundred and twenty per cent. I put myself at the service of everyone and everything. And then everything went black before my eyes: a burnout. Medical and psychiatric treatment offered little relief, and I muddled along for several years until physical complaints gradually appeared; I was constantly exhausted and doubted everything. The downward spiral I found myself in led me to a mental and physical collapse. I felt that something fundamental needed to happen to prevent a suicidal outcome. My GP repeatedly urged me to seek psychiatric help. Eventually, I agreed and was referred to a psychiatrist. After an initial consultation, a full admission to the clinical psychotherapeutic ward of a psychiatric hospital was decided upon.

My greatest expectation was to recover physically and heal psychologically so that I could function normally in society again. Admission, at the age of forty-seven, was a significant challenge. Adapting to a prescribed daily and weekly schedule and working with a group of younger fellow patients during a period of total helplessness felt unreal. The first few days were challenging and intense: I didn't know what to say, hoped I wouldn't be asked anything and felt lost. Crucial in the initial treatment phase was creating a 'lifeline' on which we had to record significant events. As the memories surfaced and were concretised on that lifeline, it became clear to me that it was primarily an external factor that lay at the root of my condition.

I was confronted with a picture of neglect: why didn't I do the sixth year of primary school? I was in a boarding school in my fifth year, and my brother attended grammar school. They had a seventh year there, so I went with my brother to grammar school. I made my first Holy Communion a year earlier than my older sister and received Confirmation a year later ... The reason is that one family celebration was enough. Until the age of fifteen, I couldn't seriously study music. For several years, I followed the music theory lessons my father gave to the members of the brass band. On the piano, I tinkered a bit on the black keys ...

Occasionally, I composed music to accompany a poem. I showed it to my father, who didn't look at it and said nothing about it. It lay on the mantel-piece and remained there. I informed him of my performance whenever I played a concert, recital or on the radio. He never showed up and said he hadn't listened or didn't feel like listening.

All this had clear consequences for developing my creativity: the piano works I composed were in keys with five flats or seven sharps. When I later presented them to my girlfriend, my wife (a professional pianist), the (correct) answer was always: that's impossible to perform in such impossible keys!

It became increasingly clear that I had lived 'unconsciously' and that my pre-ference for something was irrelevant; I had nothing to want. I also realised that everything was okay for me, all the food was delicious, I had no opinion on my clothes ... for example, I didn't know what I didn't like or what colours I pre-ferred. I will never forget the manoeuvres my parents pulled to prevent me from marrying my girlfriend; they had someone else in mind for me. Fortunately, for the first time, I decided to go against my parent's advice and get engaged to her!

After hearing many stories and reflecting, I concluded that many fellow patients struggled with the same or similar thoughts, problems and influences as mine. Step by step, I recognised myself in the many signals that came my way. In this way, without realising it, I developed insights that gradually clar-ified the confusion of thoughts, feelings and internal conflicts. The many hours we spent together in groups, whether in therapy or joint activities, created a trusting atmosphere for me. The stay, care and support were excellent. There was a good atmosphere among the patients and carers. The group feeling greatly supported me during these very uncertain times. The staff's outstanding commitment encouraged me to take further steps in the ongoing process.

A peculiar observation at the beginning was that there was no distinction between the patients and the clinic staff regarding clothing. If you addressed someone in the first few days, you couldn't tell whether it was a nurse, a psychologist, a volunteer, or a patient!

The extracurricular activities, such as cooking and creative workshops, were enriching and encouraging. On Saturday mornings, we could go to the library, which had a wide range of reading material, including poetry collections. The fitness room offered opportunities to work on your fitness; we could even go to a local swimming pool one evening a week. The varied activities repeatedly provided new challenges and encouraged you to participate actively in these different tasks. I discovered that I also have a talent for drawing.

Visits were limited in number and time. At first, I (rightly) wasn't allowed home for weekends; this was naturally difficult to accept. However, gradually, we were able to spend weekends at home. It was a huge adjustment to fall back on freedom from a structured pattern. I was always happy to return to the clinic because I experienced positive progress there. We were in safe hands there and lived in a clearly defined life pattern, which was indispensable during that period!

After two-and-a-half months of very close monitoring and having discovered a great deal, my psychiatrist concluded that I was old and wise enough to continue the process in my familiar and loving home environment, but with sufficient follow-up and contact: therapy three times a week and a consultation with the doctor every two weeks. He clarified that I still had to delve deeper into everything and that a difficult period lay ahead.

Intense fears initially dominated this long period: I went shopping with a great deal of anxiety; I dreaded the moment someone would speak to me. What should I say? Should I talk about my situation and condition? Nightmares were legion; the most improbable fears and uncertainties piled up. I felt unstable and insecure; my self-confidence was gone entirely. In conversations with my wife, it often happened that one word from a sentence was enough to make me explode! I had no idea how to react. I questioned everything and needed a consistent answer to everything. It was inhumanely hard to still believe in recovery …

Important observation: the people closest to you are confronted with all possible aspects of your instability. It is, therefore, certainly not surprising that I found that many relationships among my fellow patients broke down. The partner or loved ones must endure much and have angelic patience! I can only express my immense appreciation, respect and gratitude for their commitment and perseverance! For months, I worked for hours every day in the garden, on the earth, and in this way, I rediscovered my love for nature; I learned to see how nature constantly reinvents itself in absolute diversity and beauty!

The start of outpatient psychotherapy was difficult at first: I had no idea what I should or could say or tell; during that hour, sometimes long, painful silences fell! Doubt, fear and insecurity were rampant! Gradually, however, the situation improved.

All praise, appreciation and gratitude to my psychotherapist. She was strict but fair: a position taken after a few weeks of contradiction was not tolerated; all the elements leading to it were examined again. She made it clear to me, step by step, that everything started with myself each time and that I had to start with myself. Again and again, we delved deeper, searched, described and remedied; I realised that this was the only way to find myself again, to work correctly on my reconstruction and eventually to flourish again ...

An anecdote: after months of three sessions a week and noticeable progress, I suggested that my psychotherapist reduce the sessions to two appointments. After two weeks, I begged her to please increase it back to three contacts because I couldn't manage independently. I still desperately needed guidance, in-depth exploration and support through regular constructive conversations.

If I remember correctly, I was in treatment with my psychotherapist for at least two years, also with regular process guidance sessions with the psychiatrist. Both these people have been 'life-defining' for me. Thanks to their commitment and motivation and urging me to think, I rebuilt my life mentally, from childhood through puberty, adolescence and adulthood – this required years of adaptation, acceptance, commitment and adjustment. Even when I started teaching again, I regularly had to encourage and adjust my regained positivism.

The entire process has led me to realise only now how important it is to first and foremost know yourself to make a correct assessment of your capabilities. To know your limits, your limitations. I now realise that I have been given many opportunities and that I have unconsciously been able to and may use them for the good. As a result, a peaceful and calm feeling now predominates in my inner being. Fear is a word that is no longer in my vocabulary. Service is there if it is acceptable and justifiable to me.

One negative element remains: I still dream that I conflict with my father at least once a week. In the beginning, it was characteristic that I always tried to defend myself but could not speak correctly; it was a jumble of words that I uttered. Gradually, this disappeared, leading to escalating arguments and quarrels in which I always stood up to him and tried to get my way. Such a dream usually ends with me waking up from my shouting ... I do feel that this drains a lot of energy.

Artistically, I have interpreted this memorable past in a composition for oboe and organ entitled: 'Laesus' (= wounded). Part one: Andante is very expressive, given the penetrating timbre of the oboe. Part two, Allegro, is a driven rhythmic and melodic struggle for victory over the dark past.

In recent years, I have made rapid progress to the extent that I feel connected with the composer. In his compositions, I see the structural content, the creative method of his musical language, and the specific artistic personality that he has developed. When reading a score, I understand the language the composer speaks. Also, when performing a composition, I feel at one with the work and sense what the composer expects from the performer. This makes me happy and encourages me to gain further insights.

In my creativity as a composer, I have found my language (I had it but didn't know it ...). I firmly believe that music is a language, like spoken language, that can be recognised in the structural content of compositions. My inspiration has become almost boundless, and my ideology is already clearly outlined when writing the first version. However, physical limitations and a lack of composition training prevent me from progressing even more.

I am amazed at what my inventiveness can lead to, and I realise I had to go through this deep valley to climb to a much higher level. My task and duty were to put these achievements at the service of my many artistically gifted students as much as possible. I have been able to and may use the many opportunities satisfactorily. My future lies in this: to be grateful, to further develop my talents and to put them at the service of others to the extent still feasible for me.

30 R.B.

The third time's the charm! When something doesn't work immediately, it often does on the third attempt. This can also be used to illustrate what happened to me three times. Three represents the correct number, a nicely fitting whole picture, or completeness. It was also in the third phase that I could start speaking of a successful period: from picking myself up and moving on, from quickly getting back on my feet through self-disclosure under certain conditions to walking the path to recovery. I see a movement within this from resistance and struggle stemming from defence, ignorance and protest surrounding my problems to accepting the need for help to realising that therapy is genuinely essential for life.

My psychotherapeutic process began roughly ten years ago. I ended up in a Psychiatric Acute Care unit (PWGH) via the emergency department and intensive care after a while. I had to return there shortly after my first discharge. Following this, I was referred to a clinical psychotherapeutic ward in a psychiatric hospital (PH). The movement from PWGH to PH repeated itself three times during this period.

My progress only accelerated in that third phase. By going through the process in phases, I managed to stay afloat. I received care in a regime of residential admission, day therapy or aftercare. To this day, I still benefit from outpatient psychotherapy.

At the start of that third admission period, virtually everything had slipped from my grasp. I couldn't deal with my past correctly. The sea was stormier than ever. Sunrise coincided with sunset. The beach was a mass of quicksand. The inspiring horizon remained a thick fog day and night. I was deep below sea level. No matter how far I fled, I was always brutally overtaken. I couldn't digest my past, like a brick in my stomach. The brick only grew heavier. My symptoms increased exponentially. I had convinced myself that I could make a fresh start as if a large eraser could wipe away all traces. The more I tried to sweep my past under the rug, the more painful and numerous souvenirs surfaced. I was mentally trapped. The effects were profound. I had become very distant from myself. I constantly flirted with the limits of burnout. My creed was better, harder, faster, stronger. I found no rest anywhere or in anything. When asked how I was doing, I invariably replied: 'I'm fine, I'm fine!' My thoughts and actions always hinted at 'Oops, oops!'. My attitude: 'Whew! Keep going! Don't give in!'

Since the Monseigneur Vangheluwe affair (*M.K.*: Bruges bishop; concerning sexual abuse within the Catholic Church) came to light, the sun hasn't shone fully. The survival strategies I used were no longer working, and all my remaining mental reserves were exhausted. It was as if my history kept repeating itself in different contexts and forms. My functioning could be described as 'old wine in new bottles'. I relived my history. Anxious and gloomy feelings grew increasingly intense. At a certain point, the light went out. The extent to which I decompensated showed that an unbearable weight burdened me.

'Life must be understood backwards, but it must be lived forwards!' Søren Kierkegaard left us this legacy. Against all my expectations, and certainly against my will, my past came to light. The place where I was born, its composition and its circumstances had everything to do with the problems I was facing. No one chooses where they are born nor who first looks after them. To let new and renewed wind blow through my life, I had to look at who, how and where I first received wind in my sails. I fought against this for a long time. The resistance I experienced was immense. I couldn't believe I had to see my childhood and adolescence as a starting point for facing the future.

As a developing child and teenager, I lacked a safe and warm place and the accessibility and availability of reliable support figures. Early childhood experiences and repetitive events inflicted deep wounds. A secure attachment, therefore, lacked all foundations. This made me very wary of life. I had little to no trust in the world, let alone in myself. I was always on my guard. I was an anxious child with adult antennae who struggled with many psychosomatic complaints.

My adolescence was a complex and confusing period. There were already indications of damage and stagnation. Furthermore, I felt my different sexuality confirmed, to my shame and detriment. The lack of a home meant I sought refuge in the Catholic Church. I was already at a prestigious boarding school at a very young age. My home was only a place to sleep, wash and use the toilet during short weekends. Apart from striving for excellent school results, almost everything was focused on the church and the cross. Like an orphaned child, I sought a home with a heavenly father and an ecclesiastical mother. Within that environment, I also crossed paths with several less righteous figures in fulfilling their mission and crossing several boundaries. The severe damage done to my 'new' trust and the unpleasantness I experienced further disrupted my development. Excessive vigilance increasingly characterised me. Yet, as an adolescent, I also took a step towards a far-reaching engagement: a demanding study choice and a life commitment.

Therefore, I initially received psychotherapy with considerable resistance. I experienced much internal protest at letting people delve into my heart and mind (allowing them to) stir in that stinking pot or even lift the lid. Gaining and building trust was not easy.

I kept it bearable for myself by initially rephrasing my diagnosis as burnout: 'Taking on too much for too long!' This one-sided view of the situation made it more bearable than facing the trauma. I also became acquainted with my psychopathological diagnosis in a less-than-proper way. I received a registered letter from the insurance company informing me that I had been refused a debt settlement insurance. Due to a confluence of unfortunate circumstances, an additional medical questionnaire had to mention my first admission to that PWGH. Instead of conversing, they preferred sealed envelopes to spare me and my environment. I became even more afraid of myself and the care system.

For a long time, I kept my lips sealed. Stigma and self-stigma contributed to this. Not being taken seriously or believed was something I knew from the past. Perhaps that was even the worst, most burdensome trauma. I made myself at least partly responsible for everything that had happened. I was incredibly ashamed. I was terrified of the negative consequences if I broke my promise to remain silent. Loyalty played a significant role: 'Whoever urinates against the church is playing a dangerous game!' Dare to look at the trauma, to process it, wasn't evident for this reason, let alone looking at the trauma before the trauma.

From the prognosis regarding the duration of my stay in that hospital environment, I only remembered the first part: 'As short as possible and as long as necessary!' I felt the hot breath of society pushing me to resume work as quickly as possible, burning in my neck. Week- and month-long admission has an impact on many areas. I felt overwhelmed and this caused me to cling to familiar and trusted patterns: quick processing and escaping forward. I just wanted to continue living, preferably with as few adjustments and impact as possible, without continuing to suffer.

To overcome the trauma and my past, I had to confront it again and go through it again. Therapy requires enormous effort in this respect. Besides the effort, it costs a lot of money but, above all, much time. The time that I didn't think I had or deserved. Social pressure, financial consequences, consequences at work level and an unfavourable prognosis put time under pressure. To start the process, however, I would have to trust. It logically took longer because my basic trust had been fundamentally and repeatedly damaged. That's why I went through a phased process.

It was only during that third lengthy admission that I entirely told my story, my resistance subsided, and I gave permission for care. Talking on prescription! All other medications lacked effective action or only caused side effects. I abandoned caution and restraint to open my backpack, describe and inventory its contents, and empty it. This allowed me to make room to put other things in it along the way for my further journey.

Psychotherapy appealed to me in many different ways regarding the need to better care for the trauma, the unprocessed, by looking at it calmly together, digesting the pain and facilitating the conditions for trauma recovery:

space, time, genuine care, safety, reliability, support, professional and above all accessible help. I was given the time and space to process it all.

As a physical and precious asset, I cherish my answers in words and images to three times drawing/writing 'my tree', 'my house', 'my life as an animal' and 'my life story'. I also carefully keep all the expressive assignments, pen strokes and other therapy outcomes. In the meantime, I even find myself touched, perhaps moved, by their evolution.

The emphasis should be less on the group setting. I already found it so difficult to trust the care providers. On top of that, having a group party to share my experiences and story was no easy thing. A lot has changed in the psychotherapeutic world over the period. For the better, one is moving away from one-size-fits-all approaches. Not everything is helpful for everyone. I strongly encourage using demand-driven care and a differentiated approach via expert networks. The context is also increasingly relevant. I applaud this.

The foundations were firmly laid upon which to build further. From the ward, I was guided, even during my admission, to a beacon of experience for outpatient follow-up. Through this targeted referral, I continued psychotherapy in a psychoanalytic and dynamic way.

We started again from my story without a set timeframe. I had learned in the meantime that linking psychotherapy to time doesn't work. Unconscious emotions and thoughts were made visible to better understand and process the problems' background. My ideas and feelings were set in motion. This created greater awareness and clarification and improved relationships with others, but above all, with myself. Further focusing on insight and self-knowledge, as well as comprehending my situation, instilled peace. I learned to let questions be questions, to find peace in my unrest.

For me, this tailored care was extremely helpful. Respecting my rhythm, style and pace allowed me to continue progressing, so we opted for sustainability. I further used my introspective and reflective abilities, which increased my insight into myself and my problems. By untangling what had hurt me so much, we came to a point where I could continue further, albeit with a scar, but a scar that I treat with care.

By analytically and dynamically looking together with my psychotherapist at what could strengthen my resilience, we made the burden less heavy. The line remained open with the clinical psychotherapeutic ward (the mother clinic). I received further targeted follow-up and process guidance from this home base. By letting others think and look along as partners, growth remained possible and was even enriched.

At the right time and place, the right people gave the necessary nudge in the right direction. It also felt okay because they could assess the context within which my story took place. Their own experience, knowledge and insight supported me. They lived the words: 'You can only heal the wounds of another if you have some yourself' (Jung).

Sharing expertise, experience and knowledge creates a specific closeness. By looking and listening with present attention and empathy, it also became clear what could develop further. We reached various recovery levels or 'being in my power' degrees. Strengths increasingly came to the forefront above weaknesses: qualities and personal characteristics, talents and skills, ambitions, dreams and wishes, environmental strengths and support sources, life experience and self-knowledge. Belief in my resilience further pulled me along. This further fuelled psychic growth and self-realisation even more.

I was thus set on my way with an invitation to action that placed all responsibility on myself and started with my strengths: doing something constructive with my own experience and story. From there, I could continue working in a mode of powerful vulnerability instead of just dealing with a painful injury. Recognition, the giving of language and existence, mentalisation, normalisation and psycho-education guided me increasingly towards safer harbours. Even within the Church, no sea was too high for sincere recognition. This helped to make an even cleaner ship.

I experience the whole process as reconciliation: a kind of giving a 'kiss' to myself. I feel the effect of embracing myself in my daily thoughts, actions and feelings. Psychotherapy ensured that I increasingly stopped looking at myself and the world around me through my anxious glasses. The gradually decreasing anxiety increased my insight, curiosity, knowledge and purpose.

Such a process naturally proceeds in wave-like movements. It is never a short trip on calm seas. There was energy for steering my course in the ship's hold: pen, paper and ink … lots of ink. Photography and poetry, as well as amazement and wonder in words and images, were also helpful, as were literature and music. I now cherish these things as an expression of a reborn self.

Something else I must mention about my psychotherapeutic process: the critical contribution of ex-patients/experience-workers in a mental health care centre: it is a highly fascinating and enriching education that I am allowed to enjoy: not therapy in the form of study, but a long-term and sustainable process with a powerful therapeutic effect on further personal growth and recovery in the function of and promotion of others. This forms my path to help and care provision from within, from my experience and personally gained insight. From, and not about, my own story.

With the third time's charm, the stormy sea calmed down, and the usual ebb and flow found its way again. The surf brightened. The fog cleared, and the sun shone again, even more beautifully. It is like anchoring the sailing ship within yourself. A boat in the harbour is safe but not made for that. Gustav Jung: 'I am not what happened to me. I am what I choose to become.'

31 S.C.

A combination of factors led to my 'collapse' five years ago. Professionally, I was stuck in an exhausting and barely fulfilling job. Relationally, I had a break-up to deal with and escaped into partying and meaningless flings at weekends. As a thirty-something in a big city, I lived in a shared house, and when my female housemates simultaneously decided to move out after two years, I felt utterly lost and abandoned. I burst into tears on the floor at the news of their departure. It was an over-the-top reaction, perhaps, but I was broken. It was the last straw in a bucket overflowing for a long time. Over the years, I'd lost touch with myself, played a role in the outside world, and driven myself into the ground. A crash was inevitable.

Of course, something much deeper was at play. Therapy forced me to look back at my past. I denied the impact of a dysfunctional upbringing – 'every home has its crosses' – and I imagined myself stronger than my background. My body proved otherwise at a later stage, even psychosomatically, hyper-ventilation, panic attacks, spasms and stammering.

I had been taking an antidepressant for years and occasionally had psy-chotherapy (starting when I graduated from university when I battled a first persistent depression). After my collapse, I fled the big city, ashamed of my perceived weakness, and moved back in with my parents. In an unhelpful environment and socially isolated, it was only a matter of time before I checked myself into a hospital A&E. My mind had 'gone crazy' upstairs, the gloom and suicidal thoughts more persistent than ever. I accepted I needed urgent profes-sional help. After a six-week stay in the psychiatric acute ward, without noticeable improvement, I was referred to a clinical psychotherapeutic ward in a psychiatric hospital. The approach there was psychoanalytic, both individu-ally and in groups. Shame remained a barrier throughout my entire journey. I desperately sought a way out of my suffering but found no satisfactory solu-tion. The (at the time, in my eyes) pointlessness of the therapies made me rebellious, fuelling frustration and impatience.

I just wanted to get better as quickly as possible. Everything went incredibly slowly. Resting, relaxing, catching my breath; I couldn't manage it. On the con-trary, such advice made me even more rebellious. The perceived shame of being a psychiatric patient, a 'mad person'. The feeling that nobody understood me – although that reproach primarily concerned me: I didn't understand myself. My thoughts raced, self-destructive. I considered myself weak. Despite advice to follow a more extended treatment course, I opted for a short admission. Deter-mined to work harder than others so that my recovery would be faster – I'd show them, I told myself. It was an illusion, as it turned out; at the end of the course, I had to start again from scratch in the ward for more prolonged admissions.

I was mainly looking for a concrete solution to my breakdown, like, 'You must do this, and then it will improve.' I was prepared to lay everything on the table honestly, hoping a solution would present itself more quickly. I approached advice mainly sceptically, feeling that I already knew everything and had thought about it a thousand times. Clichés like meditation, regular sleep, healthy eating, etc., made me bristle. That patience was essential for recovery didn't occur to me.

My experience with therapy was initially mainly immense frustration. I wanted a more intensive programme; everything went incredibly slowly and remained insufficiently concrete. I remember the feeling of powerlessness: I'd rather dig a ten-metre-deep pit with my bare hands to cure myself than sit 'doing nothing' among a bunch of whiners. I hated the pathetic drama.

My head was overflowing with thoughts and self-analyses, and I wanted to give therapists an insight into this. But where to begin? An hour was over so quickly. And the next patient was already waiting in the corridor. Therapies seemed to be consistently chatting about the past, repeating what I already knew for a long time. What difference did an incident from thirty years ago make to my current situation? In the darkest moments, believing that a bit of 'associative rambling' helped to move forward was particularly difficult to accept. I resisted for a very long time and thus significantly delayed my recovery. However, I couldn't go anywhere else and had to learn the lesson willy-nilly. My extreme impatience meant I had to practise even more patience.

When breakthroughs were finally achieved during sessions, nothing concrete happened. 'Time to wrap up' – the most hated phrase from a therapist's mouth. Afterwards, they sometimes said: 'Well done!' I always thought that was nonsense. Just some chatting, what kind of work is that? And what did I do with the newly acquired insight? I wanted more, more, more! I had to learn to feel that my body was indeed tired.

The strength of group psychotherapy was the recognition of the stories of others. The feeling that there were others with similar problems. That support and connection offered comfort. But equally, I listened for an entire session to a boring monologue from some chatterbox. I couldn't stand some people; that's the same 'in the outside world'. I have learned, through trial and error, that those who get on my nerves are ultimately the most valuable. Because they trigger strong emotions, they simultaneously offer the chance to confront unpleasant feelings – an opportunity to learn to set boundaries. Most of the time, I avoided such conflicts. The thing I least wanted to talk about was the most important. That seems obvious on paper, but it was challenging in practice. Like a painful wound that you'd rather not touch, but the pus has to come out eventually. The same with 'mental dirt'. It takes a lot of courage and strength.

I suspect that the tensions were highest during the group sessions. The therapist often barely said a word, just mumbled in agreement. Firmly stirring up everyone's frustration. On the one hand, I also cursed: do you have to study for so long for that? On the other hand, I felt sympathy: what a job, always swallowing criticism from rebellious patients because you can't offer them immediate help.

It was also striking that when I mentally prepared myself to tell certain anecdotes, arguments, etc. during an individual therapy session, it turned out to be less productive. A better approach was an attitude of 'What am I going to say now?'. Then I was sometimes surprised by what suddenly came up. Surprised by my own words. The condition was to speak openly and freely, a skill I really had to learn. At first, that felt very awkward and vulnerable. I preferred to keep the embarrassing things to myself. Again: precisely that turned out to be the most relevant thing to tell. As if I was standing naked.

Sometimes a severe crisis helped. During an outburst, only genuine feelings come out. That also provided extra material to talk about afterwards. Intuitively, a person knows a lot, but filters (social, from upbringing, through trauma, etc.) prevent information from coming to the surface. Sometimes I saw what was going on with someone else, but pre-empting didn't help. That person had to realise it themselves, at the frustratingly slow pace that it requires. Speaking freely and associatively in the presence of a therapist led my mind down new paths. On my own, endlessly ruminating, I too easily fell into the same thought patterns, mainly self-condemnation.

Nowadays, I keep my eyes closed during sessions. On the one hand, to get closer to what I feel inside, on the other hand, because I don't want to see the other person's reaction. That influences me; the slightest movement or sigh generates a new stream of thoughts, and then I start projecting negatively: 'He/she finds it boring', etc. Consequently, I would adapt and be less honest.

Specific therapies and assignments drove me up the wall. Namely, occupational therapy and 'draw yourself as a tree' or 'sculpt the monster inside you' – I felt like I was in kindergarten. Or music therapy, where we all drummed on drums or danced improvisationally. Difficult to cope with. I threw myself into extracurricular sports activities like a madman. An ideal outlet for anger and powerlessness. Striving and performing to the utmost. At times, I felt like I was at a sports camp.

The actual insight that brought about a breakthrough in my recovery did not come from therapy but from a conversation with a friend. I told her unpleasant memories from my childhood and thus gained an understanding of my parents' crucial role and impact. A moment of revelation. It felt like an earthquake and was accompanied by severe panic attacks. Extremely overwhelming. My foundations were shaken.

To truly understand what happened during my childhood today, it helps to abstract the situation, distance myself and tell it as a straightforward story about a child as if it doesn't concern me. There's a photo of myself as a toddler on my mantelpiece. I then try to imagine what growing up was like for that little one. An only child, a depressed mother, a father who drank a little too much, a lot of arguing, and the child as an interpreter between both parties. The mother calls the child her 'everything', praises it to the heavens and spoils it excessively. The father is highly jealous and sidelined. The mother takes the child everywhere, like a trophy, and uses it as an excuse for secret trips to an extramarital affair. The child becomes a silent witness and accomplice in all sorts of secrets. When the child is six, the affair comes to light. The father, beside himself with rage, blames the child for keeping the secret. Despite the revelations, the unhappy marriage continues. The mother meets new lovers, and the situation continues to grow skewed. I find the psychiatrist's statement enlightening: love between parents is more important for the child's development than their love for the child.

With the help of a therapist, a strategy was developed to approach things differently and (dare) to make difficult decisions. So, I broke contact with my parents and gave myself space to process suppressed emotions such as anger and sadness. As a child, I couldn't experience them for self-preservation; as an adult, I can and must allow them to heal.

I had a year-and-a-half of clinical psychotherapy in a psychiatric hospital. First in full inpatient treatment during my worst crisis, then day therapy and finally outpatient psychotherapy. Together with a social worker, I prepared for a return to the big city – my apartment, creating a safe environment. I've come a long way, but in my opinion, therapeutic work is still ongoing.

'Recovery', in my experience, doesn't necessarily have to do with work ethic or motivation; the body dictates the pace. The fact that I didn't realise the impact of my past for so long is very telling. Unfortunately, things that I carried and suppressed for a whole life don't just get resolved. Because I wanted everything faster than prescribed, it ultimately took longer. My resistance to some therapies was also a hindrance. Through my protest, I only boycotted myself.

Knowing rationally that something was wrong in my upbringing fundamentally differs from emotionally realising it. Now, I believe you must be 'ready' to face certain truths to process them. Despite willingness, it doesn't come automatically. Even to this day, after all the therapy I've had, traumatic memories still surface, to my surprise, that I've never told anyone before. I find ignorance, those blinders to such an impactful reality, astounding.

Compared to before, I pay more attention to my own needs. Previously, I adapted to others and 'the norm' and didn't listen enough to my own body. But there's a limit to being strong and gritting your teeth. It's better to allow help; otherwise, you risk breaking.

Unpleasant feelings like sadness, anger or fear are human, and I must learn to bear them. The meditative thought helps: instead of resisting them, I might as well accept that they are there. Then, their impact diminishes. At certain moments, I doubt my sanity (after all, I was 'in psychiatry'), or I fear that it will never get better; after all, I've felt so bad for such a long and intense time, maybe depression is in my genes? I also try to accept those anxieties, like a twitch or sitting in a cramped position for too long. Then I ask myself: can I tolerate these feelings or thoughts? The answer is usually yes. That relieves the pressure and creates distance. Thoughts are just thoughts.

What has therapy given me? My first reaction was a lot of misery and tears. I learned in the hospital about the term 'mental suffering'. Naming it makes it real and distinguishes it from attention-seeking. I believe I've become stronger – 'what doesn't kill you ...'. I also experience more acceptance. More grounded. Before, I could achieve great things and change the world. Now, I try to accept my shortcomings. Pain, failure and setbacks, just like the good things, are equally part of life; there's no point running away from them – a fitting expression: the art of being unhappy.

I've had to learn to put pride aside. I'm sometimes still ashamed, as if I'm weak. However, I've learned to be more open with my surroundings about mental vulnerability. Everyone in my environment reacts understandingly, and I feel supported. I've adopted a healthier lifestyle and am more honest with myself, with precise attention to my sensitivities. My journey may deviate from what is 'usual', but so be it.

My most considerable criticism afterwards remains that long search for suitable help. Mental illnesses are inherently a delicate subject, and there's still a taboo surrounding them (fortunately, increasingly less so). Then, approaching various agencies and healthcare providers and receiving the most absurd advice or wrong diagnoses makes the process much more painful than necessary. That you then still have to have much patience during treatment, that it's expensive, and that you don't see immediate results still frustrates me.

I'm doing pretty well overall these days. After realising my traumatic past and experiencing the accompanying emotions, the next step seems to be to forgive and enter a new 'normality'. My parents certainly meant well; in a way, they are also just victims of their past. I want to understand my past and move on healthily.

How my future will concretely translate professionally, relationally, or family-wise is still a question mark. But that's true for most people. I mainly hope to continue to live honestly with myself.

32 S.J.

When my eldest daughter collapsed at the age of eighteen, I had to be strong. She told me she had been abused by her father, my ex-husband, from the age of six or seven. I went with her to the child abuse centre, the GP, and the CMHC (community mental health centre). I also wanted to go to the police with her, but she refused. It soon became apparent that she had already shut herself off and didn't want to discuss it anymore. I was left with many questions. What had he done? How far had he gone? Was it only that one daughter (I have four daughters and two sons)? I also had much guilt, and my mother only made it worse.

The CMHC and my GP felt I needed help, so I started going to the CMHC and my GP every other week. The sessions there were only about the children and my ex, not about me. Eighteen months later, the CMHC therapist felt we were stuck and referred me to a psychiatrist. Another six months later, everyone (except me) agreed: a short inpatient stay was necessary. An appointment was made for an intake interview at a short-stay adult ward in a psychiatric hospital. An eight-week stay seemed reasonable, but after two weeks, the team decided I needed longer and moved me to a different ward.

At first I felt my problems weren't serious enough for hospital admission. I was depressed and had physical symptoms, but I thought those would pass with time and a pill. I had constant terrible headaches; I couldn't tolerate any noise – my children couldn't have crisps anymore because I couldn't stand the sound;

even opening a bread bag made me cringe. I'd also lost my voice six months previously; I could only whisper, and sometimes not even that. I was practically unable to sleep and, if I did, I was guaranteed a nightmare. I couldn't work anymore (as a carer for children with multiple disabilities) because, with every child, I wondered if there was abuse in the parent-child relationship.

My biggest problem was the fact that my ex-husband abused my daughter and what my role in it was. I couldn't cope with it. I only expected to find a way to process this awful event, and I didn't think that should take eight weeks. I had never heard of psychotherapy before, so I didn't know what to expect. It didn't work at all with the psychologist. He just said nothing, and I'm not much of a talker either. During individual therapy, it was primarily silent until he'd say: 'Time's up, see you next week?' Group therapy wasn't much better. Sometimes, group members spoke, sometimes not. With the psychiatrist, however, it clicked. I trusted him almost immediately. Together, we managed to unearth the Pandora's box of traumas hidden inside me. It wasn't always pleasant, but it had to be done.

It became clear that I had been neglected from a very young age. The school and the child and adolescent mental health service intervened a couple of times, and we were placed in care twice. From the age of ten to fourteen, my father used me as a prostitute. I was forced to have sex with men, and my father was paid for it. We did a lot to get money and cigarettes, but this was by far the worst. The only relationship I ever had was with the man I married at eighteen, the father of my children. He initially seemed like my saviour, but he drank and sexually abused me in every way imaginable. He also forced me to have sex with men and couples he brought home.

In the psychiatric hospital, I learned what psychotherapy could do. I think building a bond with your psychotherapist is crucial for psychotherapy to succeed. Trust is the key to success. The sessions with the psychiatrist were both healing and confronting.

My psychotherapeutic process isn't finished yet. I'm now in outpatient therapy, but I was in full-time inpatient and day therapy for many years. It's been a long road, but there was a lot to process; it still is. Psychotherapy has changed my life a great deal. Where I used to have many feelings, anger, fear and shame, I now feel understanding. I still have the same feelings, but I now know where they come from, and it's okay that those feelings are there. It's too early for me to look to the future. I live day by day, sometimes even hour by hour.

33 T.V.

My problems started in childhood. My 'parents' never gave me any love. I suffered, and still suffer, psychologically because my mother never really wanted me. My stepfather sexually abused me. I couldn't build basic trust with these people who were supposed to 'care' for me. Yet I kept myself strong. But then, a period came in my marriage where I felt lonely. Then everything went to the surface, and it was unstoppable. I didn't want to live anymore; I had extreme and illogical fears. I fled from everything, even hidden from people. I realised I had lived with those fears all those years and never really trusted anyone. The only help I ever received was a two-week stay on a children's ward when I was eleven. I was given sedatives. They had taken me there because I refused to eat or drink. I was also terrified. After that short admission, I went back home. It was never spoken of again by anyone.

I had absolutely no expectations when I ended up in the hospital. I thought no one could help me until I met the psychiatrist, who was able to pinpoint exactly what caused all my problems. He shook my hand and said resolutely, 'I will help you'. That sentence played on my mind for a long time. One person said: 'I will help you.' A light went on for me. I believed him and was ready to accept help. It would be a long road.

At first, I found the psychotherapy unsettling and frightening. We would always have the same people in our group. If someone in my group described terrible things that a person can experience, I sometimes found it too complicated. I couldn't cope anymore and would flee from the room. I'd then have a panic attack in the corridor. They helped me with these symptoms, but I often didn't dare go back to therapy. I thought I was making a fuss. It took a long time before I dared to speak in my group myself. This was again because I didn't trust my group members. Yet, slowly, it got better. I realised that the others were my peers. My trust in the group and the therapist began to grow.

Talking about the sexual abuse was very difficult. I was ashamed of it, found it embarrassing, didn't dare. I couldn't possibly go into detail about those events, but I could talk about my feelings about them. I couldn't talk about my mother without crying. The more I told, the more it dawned on me what she had done to me. I found it very difficult to process my feelings. It felt like a grieving process, even though she was still alive.

I also started thinking differently and even became angry. Getting angry was something I'd never done. I could express that in psychotherapy. The psychotherapist was good. He sensed well whether I wanted to talk or not. The group's confidentiality outside therapy was also an excellent security for me. I think psychotherapy should stop at a certain point. You can't talk about what you've been through for your whole life.

Gradually, I grew towards a life outside the hospital. When I decided to take the next step in my life and build an everyday existence, I firmly closed the lid on that box. I can't forget, but now I can live with it.

At the beginning of my admission, group cooking or sports didn't help me. I was exhausted, and I preferred to be alone. I slept a lot, and I needed that. Once I entered everyday life, I was more interested in those activities. What also didn't help me was isolation. I experienced it once, and it made me even more agitated than before. I experienced it as punishment and felt incredibly trapped.

Other therapies did me much good: expression through drawings, dancing to music and telling my story. My personal support worker also helped me move forward. She was always there for me when things weren't going well; she caught me. Everyone involved in my recovery believed in me. They never gave up. I had ups and downs, but they kept believing in me. And I didn't give up either.

My admission lasted four years, my psychotherapeutic process lasted longer, and perhaps I'm still healing. I was thirty-two when I was admitted. Something you carry around for so long, bottle up and push away, you don't get rid of in a flash. I experienced the years in the hospital as a safe, protected environment. The only good contact in the hospital was my son. I saw him on Wednesday afternoons and at weekends. Other people were also behind me, but I lived for my son.

I still needed support afterwards when I took the step to live alone and went into co-parenting for my son. The week he wasn't with me, I couldn't cope with life and stayed in the clinic. That lasted a few months. I was thirty-six, had to reintegrate into society, and had responsibility for my son. After that, I continued with day therapy for another two years. It's not easy to build a new life, especially when you're psychologically vulnerable, but with the necessary help, my life has changed for the better.

I don't see the years of treatment as lost years but years in which I worked for myself and my child and in which I could also rebuild myself. I even became a better mother to my son. When I started the admission, I was a sitting duck. When I left the hospital, I stood firmly grounded on two feet. I overcame my fears little by little and even developed self-confidence. I deserve to be in the world and have raised my son well into a grown man without complexes and with a healthy dose of sobriety, helpfulness and empathy. He is strong in life, and I am proud of that. I am now fifty-one, and my son is twenty-four. Last year, he left home. He's doing well in life; I've done well as a mother.

For four years, I've been living with a lovely man. We didn't rush into it; we had four years of dating first. My husband understands me, also sexually. Something always remains from childhood abuse, even though I've given it a place. I have had no more contact with my mother. That's closed for me forever. My treatment saved my life; I dare say that now. I know I will need medication for the rest of my life, but that doesn't bother me.

I don't cope well with stimuli, such as shocking news images, too much hustle and bustle, and tense people. I leave people who are insincere or want to take advantage of me well alone. I have one best friend with whom I do something every week. She understands me, and we can talk nicely. I also often see my aunt, who has always supported me. We eat our sandwiches together at lunchtime. Otherwise, I like staying in my house alone with my dogs. My son and daughter-in-law also like to pop in.

I need to exercise on weekends, and I like to walk or cycle with my husband. We also have acquaintances who sometimes join us for walks. I don't need many people around me, just those I love, and that's enough. Sometimes, I still have nightmares about my mother, but I can usually put them into perspective and get on with my life. Occasionally, that doesn't work, and I don't feel well all day, but it's usually over by evening.

I find therapy very successful. I live an almost normal, ordinary life. I have come a long way with the help of nurses, therapists and my psychiatrist. If I hadn't gone into therapy, I wouldn't be here anymore.

Now I'm looking forward: I still want to go camping, have grandchildren and enjoy life's little things. Life is smiling at me, and I can now say I am a happy woman. Should something serious happen, I know I would need help again. But I also know I could pick myself up again and continue with the necessary support.

34 U.B.

I grew up in a severely psychiatrically burdened family. I have never known anything different.

My father had an untreated chronic psychiatric problem (depression, alcohol and medication addiction). Because of his unpredictable and regular outbursts, there was an atmosphere of threat at home. He was compulsorily admitted several times during periods when he posed a danger to himself and/or us. He committed suicide when I was twenty.

My mother has struggled with anorexia since the age of eleven, something that supposedly didn't exist at the time. Although her symptoms have improved significantly (relatively little underweight), the accompanying disordered eating patterns are still very prominent. I also have a younger sister who, similarly to me, has been depressed for many years and has had several hospital admissions. We both also had bulimia with an identical origin story: the first time we vomited was under my mother's coercion. She then encouraged us to continue doing this because – according to her – thin people receive more love. In terms of maternal love, this sometimes seemed to count.

My sister and I, while having similar symptomatic behaviour, coped with the situation in entirely different ways. She blamed our mother and used her for everything. I blamed myself and withdrew. My mother dealt with this situation by escaping into her career, complemented by denial of the problematic situation.

I have always had difficulties, or at least as far back as my memory goes. Since I was a toddler, I felt 'different': I was convinced I was a bad child and was regularly anxious that others would notice this and reject me. I quickly learned not to ask for help. If I tried to talk about how I felt, my mother would immediately interrupt by saying that I was ungrateful and attention-seeking and that she was the only one suffering from the situation. For me, this was reality because parents always tell the truth, don't they? So, I continued to suffer in silence.

Over the years, my depressive thoughts and anxieties grew increasingly severe. By the age of fourteen, I could barely face people; still because of that same, but even more potent, feeling: I was terrible and became convinced that people on the street saw this, that their dogs smelled it and would, therefore, attack me. Over time, I developed various ways to make my life slightly less unbearable. I started cutting myself to 'harden' myself as self-treatment against my attention-seeking behaviour. The thought that the situation wasn't endless because I planned to 'stop' my life soon gave me some courage.

Eating (albeit followed by vomiting) also brought me comfort because it put my thoughts on hold for a while. However, I became increasingly entangled in my destructive thought patterns and finally collapsed at the age of fifteen. Although I was crying incessantly, I still went to school for two weeks in that state. I spent my day in an empty classroom because it wasn't feasible for me to sit in class. Sometimes, the supervisor would come to see how I was. Through her, I contacted the CMHC (community mental health centre). From there, I was immediately referred to a child psychiatrist. Because of my increased suicide risk, she decided that admission was necessary, and I was expected the next day with my belongings. This was, however, under mild protest from my mother, whereupon the psychiatrist confronted her with the facts.

A six-week admission period was started. I genuinely believed those six weeks were sufficient to transform me into a happy, average girl. This was because I had nothing but an inaccurate picture of what was wrong with me, let alone understand its seriousness. I had internalised my mother's words: there was no problem; I just had to stop being attention-seeking. After six weeks – I wasn't happy yet – I was only poorer by an illusion. The concrete expectations of improvement with which I had begun my treatment tipped into feelings of hopelessness and despair.

The six weeks became months and eventually four years. This period consisted of a series of referrals. Each time, I was told that I had already completed the treatment plan once or several times and that they could do nothing more for me, but ... maybe somewhere else could. It created an atmosphere of unpredictability for me. Moreover, I experienced it as a kind of punishment and, therefore, as unjust. As I experienced more referrals, I cooperated less or intentionally did things wrong. In that way, I still had some control over what awaited me and when. My mother, on the other hand, sometimes found this somewhat comical. She then called me 'the boomerang' because I kept going back and forth between different services, and they couldn't get rid of me. It also made it less of a personal failure for her as a mother.

In most wards, the focus was very strongly on the binge eating I had, as this was the most visible problem: the frequency continued to increase, as did the quantities I ate. The reasoning behind this was that if the binge eating were gone, the problem would also be (essentially) solved. In my perception, this strategy came across as: if we take away the only thing that still keeps you going, then we're on the right track (needless to mention, I was very resistant to this approach).

Based on that focus on the eating problem, I was admitted twice for six months to (read: referred to) an eating disorder ward. The first time, I was almost wholly binge-free during my entire admission but very anxious, depressed and withdrawn. The second time was about three years later. At that time, I had about five binge-eating episodes per day. I only had two binge-eating episodes in the first week (instead of about thirty-five) and was proud of myself. I thought I had achieved an incredible feat. Until I mentioned this and received a dismissive reply: 'That should be better because everyone else in the group can do it without it.'

I wasted the rest of that six-month admission after that: from then on, I put all my effort into maintaining the appearance of being a 'good' patient, a 'good' child. Even though I continued to have daily binge-eating episodes in the toilets several wards away, hiding it at least meant they were satisfied with me: 'You're doing very well!'

In group therapy, the emphasis was on (symptom) behaviour: conversations were almost exclusively about topics such as who had dared to eat their chips that afternoon or who was behind schedule with their weight. In other words, it was about anything but the essence: the content of a problem did not extend beyond what you saw. To tackle the problem, we worked with an 'alternatives list': What can I do when things are bad? A crossword puzzle? Take a bath? Call mum or dad? Individual sessions revolved around the extent to which we had been able to use this list in case of difficulties.

One therapeutic approach that has stayed with me enormously was that of a ward for personality disorders, praised for its excellent results. The idea here was that you made progress by correcting (punishing) behaviour that they considered wrong. For example, if you hadn't made your bed by eight o'clock in the morning, you wouldn't get a blanket that night. If you cut yourself, you wouldn't get a personal conversation for twenty-four hours. The latter almost motivated me to cut myself because it was the ideal way to avoid talking (there didn't even have to be a conversation about why you didn't want to speak).

A pitfall of that therapy was based on the reasoning that everyone does everything for the same reason. After about four weeks, I was shown the door with the message that I first had to do something about binge eating and cutting before I was welcome back. The only thing I felt was relief. A reflection I make on this outcome is that my compulsory discharge was motivated by (the severity of) symptoms that are characteristic of the personality disorder in which that ward supposedly 'specialised'.

Indeed, people will have been helped by the therapeutic orientation of the wards where I stayed for the first four years, but unfortunately, I was not one of them. Was it because of the therapy? No. Was it because of me? For a long time, I answered 'yes' to this because I was (and am) of the opinion that in psychotherapy, the most significant responsibility ultimately lies with yourself. However, I can now nuance the image of myself as the main culprit somewhat, and I think it was more a mismatch between the therapeutic approaches I had tried up to then and myself.

I have ultimately had about ten admissions in several different places. In connection with this, I have also had experience with various types and forms of therapy: classical behavioural therapy, cognitive behavioural therapy, dialectical behavioural therapy, family therapy, group therapy, individual psychotherapy ...

The decisions to refer me were partly based on the idea that another psychotherapeutic approach might be more suitable (and, therefore, a match) for me. They were mostly made with the best intentions but not the best for me. I experienced this as a constant repetition of the feelings of rejection that characterised my childhood, a reaffirmation of my idea that I was terrible. I couldn't settle anywhere; I didn't feel at home in the sense of 'safe': accepted, not having to be on my guard against unexpected danger, as in my childhood.

There were also two 'compulsory discharges', as they were called then. I owe those entirely to myself, of course.

Throughout these four years of admissions, my anxiety decreased. Still, my self-destructive behaviour (including binge eating and vomiting) had significantly increased: I ate until I had difficulty breathing and my legs turned purple. It was the only way to stop my feelings and thoughts, which would otherwise feel unbearable. And the sense of bursting was so intense that it overwhelmed everything. So, it seemed that I had created the 'solution' rather than psychotherapy having anything to do with it. I also had the impression that I had reached the ceiling of what psychotherapy could offer me.

My mother also contributed to the low hope in therapy: at times when I expressed that I could change, that I could get better, she sometimes said: 'Just give up. They can't help you anyway; they've already proven that.' Therefore, I decided to continue outpatient treatment at a low frequency. After doing this for a year, I – at the age of majority – agreed for the first time to be admitted myself.

Since I was nineteen, I had to make the transition from a child psychiatrist to an adult one. The psychotherapy I received here differed in several respects from the therapies I had been exposed to until then.

What made the most significant difference for me is that this last clinical psychotherapeutic admission did not end in a third compulsory discharge. Not only because I could then continue my treatment but because, for the first time, there was someone who looked beyond my behaviour, who didn't send me away, who stayed behind me. Even when the entire team was indignant and, above all, dumbfounded.

There was also no such thing as 'wrong' thoughts. Free speaking (free association) was central here. Because of the non-judgemental way the psychiatrist listened, I dared to express my true thoughts for the first time. The words were sought together, and I got stuck in my thoughts. I was not used to being allowed to say what I thought: not with my mother, who silenced me, and neither in previous psychotherapies, where my thoughts were called 'wrong'. My binge eating had the same function: not thinking and especially not speaking.

Furthermore, decisions were no longer made on my behalf about what was 'good' for me. I was no longer implicitly told that I could not choose. There was no ideal to strive for and, therefore, no expectations to meet. It removed the possibility of disappointing others and being rejected. Yet I had to get used to the fact that I no longer had a point of reference about who I was supposed to be because I had adapted all my life: as a child, I twisted myself into all kinds of knots at the whims of my parents, trying to be liked. Even during the first five years of psychotherapy, I conformed to therapeutic expectations.

These differences from previous therapies meant I gradually gained confidence in the therapist. I suspect this trust distinguishes the last twelve years (one year residential and eleven years once a week outpatient) from the first five years. That trust was necessary for me to dare to show who I was, to learn to speak and, therefore, to start my therapy.

Looking back, I can only see an enormous positive evolution. It has cost me a lot of time and effort, but I never expected to reach where I am now. I don't yet know where my therapy will take me. There is no such thing as an actual endpoint, a concrete goal. There is no yardstick for progress. Often, my progress was so slow and steady that I thought I was standing still. At those times, it came down to being able to trust my therapist's judgement and accept what he said about it. I hope to close this chapter of psychotherapy, which has already taken up more than half of my life, by the time he retires.

35 V.A.

In my early twenties, a failing relationship and a dream job that became a disappointment first shook my foundations. My first depression manifested, although looking back, there were also depressive episodes during my adolescence. A psychiatrist prescribed antidepressants and referred me for psychotherapy. It helped me climb out of the pit within six months, albeit not without a price. I changed jobs, and the relationship ended.

Life resumed. The new job suited me much better. I met a new partner, whom I married and had children with. Externally, I had recovered well, but unbeknownst to the outside world, a similar dependence on my therapist developed, mirroring my earlier dependence on my parents and my first partner.

This dependence increased, gradually undermining my ability to function normally, eventually becoming unsustainable. The therapy itself had become the primary source of suffering. Ending the sessions was problematic; I constantly sought contact with my therapist, and breaks due to holidays caused panic and despair.

Too late, I managed to extricate myself from this unbearable therapy and sought help from another therapist. By then, my decline had begun. Increasing compulsiveness foreshadowed what was to come. When the same dependence pattern almost immediately repeated with the new therapist, they responded appropriately by setting boundaries. These boundaries broke me. Raw fear overwhelmed the obsessive thoughts and actions, immediately disrupting my daily life.

After two months of sick leave, I gradually returned to work. Looking back, it would have been better if I hadn't. It was a constant struggle to keep myself going and avoid collapsing into a terrifying, obscure emptiness. I tried hard to appear 'normal', yet I constantly felt that others could see right through me. Half a day's work, with a limited workload, was enough to exhaust me physically and mentally. When my father was diagnosed with incurable cancer three months later, I fell back through the fragile ice. This time, hospitalisation was unavoidable.

With my mind blank, just to overcome the taboo and shame, I admitted myself to a PWGH ward (psychiatric acute admission unit). After two weeks, I was transferred to a psychiatric hospital. The therapy programme comprised three group sessions, supplemented by sports, occupational therapy, music, a creative workshop and various elective treatments. The therapy provided structure and helped me get through the day. Meanwhile, the ongoing mental health difficulties had also put my marriage on the rocks. I was utterly lost.

My stay in the hospital was a months-long battle against overwhelming depression and moments of raw fear. An exhausting, hopeless struggle where despair and helplessness went hand in hand. Nothing seemed to help, no matter what I did. Obsessive thoughts and actions were also omnipresent. The day was a succession of unbearable, intrusive thoughts that had to be neutralised by equally absurd and shameful actions.

I desperately clung to every moment of speaking, assuming that this was where the difference had to be made. It shames me to look back at the person I was then. In group therapy, I would intrusively and excessively take the floor, hoping to voice the unspoken.

Meanwhile, the uncertainty about the survival of my marriage persisted. I went home at weekends and tried to keep going. The atmosphere at home was heavy and charged, difficult to bear – a tense fear of saying the wrong word, causing my marriage to collapse definitively. Only in the evenings did the depression somewhat lift; the obligation to get through the day was no longer present.

It's difficult to pinpoint the exact turning point in my treatment or the lever that led to recovery. I can confirm what the psychiatrist aptly said at the time: more than outpatient therapy, residential admission offers the added benefit of a caring 'mothering environment'. The hospital was a protective shell that shielded me from daily life, a life I could no longer cope with.

The question of where exactly things went wrong has been revisited many times. The cause will undoubtedly have been multi-faceted. I attribute it to insufficiently thorough individuation or not becoming sufficiently independent from my parents and others. The origin of my problems dates back to a time long before my birth. My mother was given a first name that referred to her mother's great love. A father who never wanted to acknowledge her. The taboo and shame of being an illegitimate child overshadowed my mother's entire life. The unspoken secret marked her and, by extension, me.

Being herself, simply finding a place amongst others, was never easy for her. Her individuality was constantly stifled, and the price was paid in our family. My father also had his vulnerabilities, unlike his older siblings. Did the somewhat sudden death of an older brother play a part? It shook the family to its foundations in the middle of wartime and must have drastically affected the relationships within the family. In contrast to the robust characters of my uncle and aunt, my father was somewhat fragile, timid and lacked a strong sense of self and personality, never truly separating himself from his parents.

Serious psychological problems and hospitalisation had previously prevented my mother from fulfilling her desire to have children. I was born only after twelve years of marriage. Her psychological vulnerability was also the reason why there was no second child. My parents, probably each from their experienced insecurity, found a haven in each other. It was a relationship where they didn't see the proper distance from each other and even less the appropriate space for a child to grow up.

My childhood evokes warm memories of the many visits to my paternal grandparents. But after each visit, I wondered if my mother had said the wrong thing. This was not the case, even when I thought everything had gone well. My mother didn't get along with her brother-in-law but didn't let him see it. Only at home did she express her displeasure because my father hadn't stood up for her. Again, he remained submissive and failed to meet her needs or defend himself. For my mother, his inability was always the trigger for days of stubborn silence. 'Cold wars'; I was in the middle as a child. Initially full of sympathy for my mother, later angry at her for causing yet more trouble at home, and then angry at my father for remaining helpless and powerless.

The suffocating home environment and insecurity led to psychological difficulties at a young age. At the age of nine, I had severe sleep disorders that lasted until my adolescence. The fact that it was the threat of being sent to boarding school by the doctor that brought about a change is significant and confirms my separation and abandonment anxiety as a core problem.

My long-term hospitalisation revolved around the challenging transition to standing on my own two feet. A process of relinquishing the help of others. A path that no one could pave for me. No beautiful, stylised or well-thought-out plan. I had to literally 'sweat out' that dependence, simply taking the required time. This time, the safety of the hospital and the therapeutic programme were supportive and meaningful. The neuroleptics probably also played a significant role in keeping the madness within me manageable. Like a desperate person grasping at anything to stay afloat, I eagerly availed myself of the elective therapies. I learned about relaxation, meditation, music and dance, art and creativity.

The downside of my runaway compulsiveness paradoxically kept me going. Was it determination, perseverance against better judgement, fighting spirit or discipline, or animal instinct for survival? The persistent, desperate clinging – to avoid stopping – characterised me throughout my hospitalisation and helped me through.

The step towards a little more independence for adult life seems small in retrospect, no more than crossing a thin line and paradoxical. Surrounded, not without others, yet essentially a step I had to take entirely alone. Despite the involvement of many therapists, the dominant feeling during my hospitalisation remained one of loneliness. A perception primarily coloured by my helplessness and despair.

My recovery took over a year-and-a-half – quite long and gruelling. But it involved the essential step of individuation for every human being – a process that transcends the purely conscious and cognitive and cannot simply be learned. Only time and the lack of escape routes or lifelines to cling to forced me into that painful, seemingly endless process of relinquishment.

After three months of full-time inpatient care and nine months of day treatment, I resumed my job part-time. That went better than expected. After a month of progressive employment, I returned to full-time work. Follow-up was arranged with the hospital in the form of a weekly return visit. After three months, I closed the hospital door behind me.

I could finally resume my life. Although my relationship had long been hanging by a thread, we climbed out of that valley as a couple. We have grown closer together and become more intimate. My wife now has a husband who stands more on his two feet.

The balance sheet of my crisis is undoubtedly positive, even though I suffered terribly. The childish dependence has been overcome, enabling me to lead a more normal adult life. I still see a psychotherapist, and those sessions are vital to me. But, unlike before, I no longer contact him between sessions, and the cancellation of a session is not a drama.

Professionally, as a care worker, I have become more balanced. My way of working is more refined and mature, and I no longer fanatically adhere to the letter of the theory. I need a more pragmatic approach shaped by my life experience, albeit always aware of my subjective perspective. I can take a punch better and handle much more work than before.

Besides the question of what fundamental work needed to be done, the question of how I could have deteriorated so severely despite outpatient therapy continued to gnaw at me. Responsibility for the derailment is shared.

After my first depression, I had sworn a solemn oath to investigate the cause of my breakdown thoroughly. Thoroughly investigating something is not bad as long as you remain mindful of its limitations. Who ultimately has to solve the problem, the therapist or yourself? Is it even possible to fully understand the genesis of a problem?

For a long time, I had focused all my hope and effort on therapeutic work in the narrow sense. Between sessions, I lived life as if in a waiting room. I lived from session to session, and problems that arose were postponed until the next session with my therapist. I put my fate in his hands. This was a misconception that further fuelled the existing dependence.

Let that be an essential lesson for me since then. Therapy is never limited to the therapist's consulting room. The important thing now is to get on with life. You are responsible for how you fill that life. No one can choose or decide for you. Moreover, there are no guarantees. Things can go wrong, and you have to deal with that.

I said I shared responsibility. What was the therapist's part then? Somewhere, he nurtured the delusion that my problem could be solved in therapy, or at the least, he didn't sufficiently counter it. The belief that your therapist possesses the knowledge to solve your problem is a significant mechanism that determines the effectiveness of therapy. However, this belief had taken on mythical proportions for me, having a counterproductive, paralysing effect on the therapeutic process. My concern about the increased tension and dependence was soothed by misplaced trust. A firmer setting of boundaries regarding the sessions themselves, as well as my contacts in between, would have prevented the therapy from derailing so severely.

My mental health difficulties, now over ten years ago, were the turning point in my life. A harrowing and intense period. A crisis that was unavoidable and necessary to make a different life possible. My vulnerability hasn't disappeared. I remain a restless soul whose thoughts never cease. The feeling of insecurity is never completely gone. I remain sensitive to what others think and say; too often, still too much. And the answer to the question of why I try so hard to prove myself is also easy to find. Being content with who I am and accepting things as they are without constantly questioning everything remains a challenge. Setting boundaries for myself or others, accepting limits, and dealing with anger are themes I am not yet finished with today.

And yet, I am happy with who I am and the personality my winding path has shaped. It has mainly shaped me into the competent care worker I am today. I've often said it jokingly: I didn't learn my job at school but from a young age in my home situation. My alertness to the slightest signal, both verbal and non-verbal, and my skill in navigating words and actions are excellent skills in supporting other people in their search for themselves. I now stand differently and more confidently in life. That life remains unpredictable and will continue to have its ups and downs. But I enjoy it, the big and small things. I am doing well.

36 V.B.

Just before my thirtieth birthday, I made my first suicide attempt. Many more followed. I was in a very dark place and only thought about death. I didn't know why, and the attempts were severe. I existed but didn't really 'know' anything anymore … I thought things would never get better. I lacked self-awareness regarding my illness; I just wanted to leave, to 'disappear'. I didn't know what made it so difficult; it just was. I'd struggled with suicidal thoughts since I was thirteen. Shortly before my first attempt, I was verbally abusive towards those closest to me. With others, however, there was 'nothing wrong' … I couldn't live with myself anymore. I didn't like myself. The only things I did were work, eat and try to sleep …

After my first attempt, I was admitted to a psychiatric assessment unit (PWGH) for two months. They couldn't provide me with therapy there; I was too unstable and fragile … They didn't know how to help me, so they transferred me to a psychiatric hospital. I didn't choose this; it just happened … I was like a zombie, anxiously and depressively sitting in my room. Before and at the beginning of my admission, I didn't ask for help. I just carried on, on autopilot. Before my first attempt (I worked as a nurse), I didn't know how to proceed. I sat in the waiting room of the psychologist at work several times. But every time she opened the door, I left. At one point, I took medication from work home with me. It had all become too much; I couldn't cope anymore, and I was utterly exhausted. Only when I was in the psychiatric hospital did psychotherapy begin.

The last time I was at home, I felt misunderstood and had no zest for life. But I didn't understand myself either. The only thing I knew then was that I wanted to die. I felt incredibly alone, lonely, and like I no longer belonged to society. And I was, as it were, afraid of my own shadow. Inside me, things were exploding more and more. I was furious at everything and everyone, especially myself, but nobody noticed ...

I was drained but couldn't sleep. Later, I learned that the 'inability to sleep' showed that I didn't dare to relinquish control. Before my first attempt, almost nothing showed; I could 'chat' very well but not 'speak'. All I wanted was to be freed from this terrible pain ...

I couldn't have a relationship either. I didn't let anyone get too close, literally and figuratively ... I also felt incredibly lonely, but I was afraid of being hurt. I didn't know who I could trust, so I trusted no one ...

I had no expectations of the treatment and admission. I thought I was beyond saving. I just was. I attended therapies because I had to; I later found them challenging to follow. It was hard. Later, I knew something had to change, that things couldn't go on like this, that it wasn't liveable. And that it had to come from me, too. And, if they couldn't even help me, I was utterly lost.

Psychotherapy was entirely new for me. I didn't know anyone who had had such treatment before. At first, I didn't understand it; I just went through the motions. During group psychotherapy, I kept talking to myself: 'I'll say it, I don't dare, I must, I can't, I can't get anything out ...' I couldn't breathe; a vast, deep, painful sob. Everyone looked at me, and then it was gone ... It took a long time before I said anything. And when I could manage a little, it was quiet, unclear, short, and didn't flow ...

After a while, I started to understand things a little better. And not just from what I said. I also listened to others, recognising myself in some things or not ... I started to put words to what was inside me, to what I felt.

Sharing usually made the burden lighter. But sometimes not. It wasn't easy to speak in a group. I also did much individual therapy. Sometimes, discussing things individually and then in a group was better. But some things I couldn't bring up in the group. I also kept things to myself. Things I couldn't even discuss with the therapist. My psychiatrist once told me: 'Let your demons see the light of day, and they will disappear.'

I gained insights into what was happening now and where it came from. That's how I gained insight into why I was so afraid of others and didn't let anyone get close, literally and figuratively – namely, childhood sexual abuse. I also lacked basic trust at home and, therefore, in my later life. I didn't know who I could trust, and consequently trusted no one ... I didn't know if anyone had good intentions towards me. After much therapy, I now have 'ground under my feet'.

At first, I didn't understand my psychotherapist; sometimes, I didn't know what she wanted, what she meant, and what she was showing me. After a long time, I developed a bond with her. But it could also sometimes explode between us. I also expected her to show who she was, not just as a therapist but also as a person. What I wanted then was for her to tell me whether she liked me as a person or not. She also showed her human side. For example, when I was in isolation, she would come to me to calm me down – just being there for me. Sometimes, she looked stern. Then I was afraid. I was cautious, wondering who she was. Later, when I knew her better, it went much better.

Interaction in the group was complicated. In my thoughts, they weren't there. But sometimes, it was good that it was in a group, and you learned from each other. The feedback from the therapist was critical; it sometimes stimulated me, mostly positively but sometimes negatively, and that kept me going ... This also meant I didn't feel like I was talking to walls.

At first, it was mainly about finding (inner) peace again. During this time, I hardly spoke anymore. I had to find my way in 'psychiatry'. During psychotherapy and other group therapies, I also listened to what others brought up. That's how the search for my own story began. After a while, it also came to the surface for me. But it wasn't easy to put it into words ... but I also learned from others. Sometimes, it exploded inside me. The main fuse blew, and all the lights went out ...

What was also crucial for me was that I was given the time (years) to get through it. Because of the insights, I felt less 'weird' in society, and after a long time, I dared to have conversations in the hospital and outside. The fear gradually diminished. It did me good. I got ground under my feet. Medication and other therapies were also crucial to me. Expressive therapies, for example, taught me to express myself, to find words ... Group therapies were suitable. It stimulated me to interact 'with others'. Both positively and negatively.

At first, I couldn't go outside for a long time. For my safety. I wandered through the corridors, didn't know where I was. I couldn't think anymore. I was also very suicidal. Gradually, I was allowed to go home for weekends. This stimulated my connection with my environment. That wasn't always easy. Later, in day therapy, I was encouraged to go outside more. Sometimes that wasn't easy. During this daycare, I could discuss things I had experienced outside the hospital that were difficult to discuss in therapy. In this way, I received guidance and was encouraged where necessary.

Sometimes, the pace was slowed down, and a step back was taken to move forward again. That's how everything went: day therapy, admission, and after-care, all intertwined. Support outside the hospital was also arranged. So I lived in supported housing for a while, then moved on to the mobile team, family support and sessions with the psychiatrist ... And sometimes, depending on my progress, these were used if things weren't going so well, and then again, okay ...

At the final stages of my intensive treatment, I agreed with the psychiatrist to stop psychotherapy, that it was complete. Psychotherapy has been essential for me. I gained insights, and I knew what had happened and what was happening. But this therapy is finite. At a certain point, I then moved on to a psychosocial rehabilitation ward. There, I learned how to react to certain situations appropriately. For others and myself. In both negative and positive situations. After much effort, it also started to work better.

I've now been discharged for six years. The support outside the hospital has become less intensive. I still see my psychiatrist regularly on an outpatient basis. Mainly to see how I'm doing. Process supervision. There are still tricky moments, but they have been significantly reduced. However, what I also find very important is that complex things are discussed. But not only that ... sharing the positive is also very important! And I know that if, for any reason, things aren't going well, I can go to the doctor.

Because I now do experiential work in the same hospital and feel it would be difficult to be admitted there, arrangements have been made. So we looked for another solution. Just knowing all this helps, and it takes away my fear. The chance of re-admission is minimal, but knowing is already a big part of the difficulty.

What has changed in me, what it has brought, is mainly that I understand myself better and where it comes from. I no longer find myself so 'weird'. I have learned from difficult, abnormal and very ordinary situations to cope with them in a standard, okay way. I'm also less afraid of people. I now dare to have a normal conversation without feeling I must tell everything. I have learned how and why 'the other' reacts like that, what is meant and why. (Mentalising: very important.) I have changed a lot during and because of the therapy. But this continues even now. This is by reacting in a certain way, continuing to build and dealing with myself and my thinking. I have become more self-confident; I no longer beat myself up. And I can now really get angry, and not just at myself. The lights don't go out anymore when I'm angry. I can handle it. I show anger and say what I do or don't think!

It all went very slowly for me! It has demanded a lot from me and still does. But I needed this time. I am incredibly grateful that this was and is possible. If I hadn't been given this time, I couldn't have done what I'm doing now: moving on. I've had many opportunities! If I hadn't received them, I wouldn't be here anymore! I now have insights, and I now know what the problems are. Now, I have learned to cope with them in as 'normal' a way as possible.

I followed psychotherapy for a long time (years), a very long road. But I think psychotherapy has an endpoint. But I know that if it were necessary again, I would go for it again. I now have such a nice, calm result. I still go for regular outpatient consultations with my psychiatrist, and I still find it necessary to vent now and then. And I also find it safe. Someone is watching over me.

How do I see the future? I can usually enjoy myself now. I now have a zest for life, something I didn't know before. It does me good. I know I must regularly check in with myself: is everything okay? And then I'm back on track. I hardly have any suicidal thoughts anymore. I can live with myself more, and I have respect for myself. In that way, it's manageable. But I sometimes fear that it might return. Even though I know I wouldn't let it get that far again. And I know there is help and how to reach it.

I haven't been admitted for six years now, and it feels safe – everything above thirty I owe to the treatment. I've never been so well. It's not always roses. No, certainly not. But for the state I'm in now, I'm very grateful. I can live freely, with fewer fears (especially social ones). I can sleep. I dare to speak. And sometimes to groups of sixty people as an experiential expert. I now do experiential work in the hospital where I was admitted before. It is suitable for me to pass on what I have received and experienced to others and my patients. I try to share as much as possible to help others. And that's working reasonably well. I try to be an added value for my patients. And it's a win-win situation. That's how I have a social job again (I used to be a nurse). That's how I feel. I *mean* something …

37 V.M.

My life didn't exactly start rosy, if I'm honest. The inspiration for my name came from a funeral card. I was also an accident: my mum took her contraceptive pill with a gulp of water from the bottle. A few pills remained at the bottom … Considering my brother was ten years older, and my parents didn't want any more children, they even considered an abortion. And as if fate wanted to intervene, I was put in the wrong crib at birth. But ultimately, I ended up where I was meant to be …

I remember very little of my early childhood. I was apparently sweet, compliant and always at the service of others. Looking back, I feel I only existed when someone looked at me. And I worked hard for that, to be seen, by behaving as exemplarily as possible. Not so bizarre, perhaps, given that my brother couldn't stand me. I was the one who knocked him off his teenage throne. I was a spoiled princess in his eyes, and I could do nothing right. He hated having to babysit me. He made things difficult for my parents during his teenage years. He pushed every boundary he could find. My father came from a large family with an authoritarian, heavy-handed father. So, my brother's antics met with more than just resistance. My brother quickly married to escape home; he was twenty-one.

From the age of twelve, I was an 'only' child at home. I knew the rules I had to abide by to avoid my father's harsh hand. And honestly, I did that brilliantly. It's as if it was ingrained in me from birth. I didn't even try: I was the princess, the angel. Being a late arrival, I never really had peers around me. I just went everywhere my parents went. I had no hobbies and wasn't in any clubs. Even my neighbours didn't have young children anymore. I was self-reliant: I played with Lego and Barbie and drew a lot.

My mother worked in Brussels, had to leave early by train and only came home late. Despite the early hours, our breakfast and lunch sandwiches for my father and me were already prepared. My father did odd jobs at weekends as a *maître d'hôtel*. This often led to arguments between my mum and dad. My mum was incredibly jealous: she checked the mileage on the car and even sniffed his shirt ... She once told me that my father had had an extramarital affair. I once received a phone call from an angry man who shouted that my father should stay away from his wife ... My father denied it then, and I never told my mother.

I chose the Latin-modern languages classes because my classmates were doing it. Despite the advice of the careers guidance counsellor, I wanted to prove that I could do it by studying hard and a lot. I was strict with myself; I couldn't score less than seventy per cent. Unfortunately, I didn't score any more either. I clung to one friend every year, but they always let me down. I often felt like the fifth wheel on the carriage in secondary school. I didn't belong anywhere: I was never drunk, didn't smoke, and didn't have a boyfriend. I often cried myself to sleep at parties. It felt like I was invisible. I was only good as a shoulder to cry on or resolve arguments. It never occurred to me to share this sadness with my parents. I wrote down my misery in a diary. During this dark period, my doctor told me that 'it' was all in my head. A statement that will always stay with me.

When I went to university, I desperately longed for a boyfriend. So much so that it hurt; I decided to study clinical psychology, hoping I might find answers to my unhappiness. The studies were again a (far too) heavy burden! Blood, sweat and tears it cost me. I often wanted to give up, but that was without my mum's knowledge. She knew my timetable better than I did. And as soon as my last class finished, the central heating in my room was already on, ready for studying. When I failed an exam, she couldn't understand why a friend's daughter had passed, and I hadn't when that daughter had only done technical subjects, and I had done Latin. During the exam period, because of exam anxiety and a mild form of self-harm, I saw a psychologist a few times. But because I didn't know what to expect and due to the far too short treatment (no click), I only managed to muddle through ... nothing more, nothing less. The unspoken pressure from my mum did help me get my degree.

Halfway through my studies, I met my boyfriend through a mutual acquaintance. He fell head over heels for me and courted me extensively. He wasn't my type, but no one had ever put so much effort into me; no one had ever looked at me like that. And I succumbed ... even more ... in a short time, he became my 'everything'. When I left home, my mum cried buckets of tears. She couldn't accept her daughter leaving the nest. Around the same time, my grandmother died, my last grandparent. I loved her very much, and with her, the whole family on my father's side fell apart. I tried everything to mend the rift to no avail. Goodbye grandmother, goodbye family ...

Luckily, my boyfriend was my soulmate; we did almost everything together, and I could even finish his sentences. Everything seemed to be going smoothly, I thought. But even during that period, my parents continued to have more influence on me than I realised. We still went everywhere with them. In my eyes, that just showed my good relationship with them. My mum came to clean when I was pregnant, lovely! But after every cleaning, our belongings were always in a different place. And that's something she still does; she leaves her mark everywhere ... She also often says (unsolicited), 'If you ask me, I would do it like this. But you do what you want, of course.' Usually, I did it her way, the only 'right' way ...

History repeated itself with my brother and me: I gave birth to a (too) compliant angelic daughter and four years later to a very strong-willed son. After his birth, an unhappy feeling slowly awoke (again?). My boyfriend's attention, which had once been solely for me, now had to be shared with three. My daughter's constant crying and my son's constantly pushing boundaries meant my energy levels were dropping. When my son was four, completely distraught, I tried to get a grip on myself through therapy, on my outbursts and my (known) feeling of not being seen. Because one thing I was sure of, I was the problem: I was failing on all fronts: as a partner, mother, daughter, sister and friend ... When my boyfriend decided on Valentine's Day ten years ago that I didn't need to come home anymore, I ended up in the hospital psychiatric ward. The psychiatrist on duty referred me after a few months to a psychiatric hospital (often called 'mother' P.). This clinic became my safety net, a time for respite and recovery. For six months, I had the chance to catch my breath to see that there was (still) something to live for. The combination of therapists, nurses, care and fellow patients gave me the strength to try again. Thanks to a phased return to work, I started working again. My children needed a mother, and I wanted a new relationship. During that time, my quest to find myself began ... with many falls and rises. I tried to go against my parents for the first time but paid dearly for it. To this day, I'm told that I broke my mother's heart.

Acupuncture, osteopathy, behavioural therapy and coaching therapy – nothing I didn't try. Money flowed freely, but the feeling of well-being remained absent. I also tried to alleviate my inner pain with alcohol.

Due to a merger at work (where my beloved counter job disappeared) and another failed date, I started a second course of treatment at P. three years ago. This time, I wanted to dig deeper, understand why and where I always backed out, and expose my roots. Frustratingly, my psychiatrist indicated that therapy in psychiatry only comprises a part of the process and that the most prominent part would take place outside the protective walls/arms of the hospital. So, after a short course in the hospital, I started an outpatient course with weekly therapy. And honestly ... this was a wise choice! All the therapeutic and other help before had only allowed me to stay afloat. The weekly treatment with the psychiatrist, thankfully, goes further. During our sessions, I'm learning to see that much of my insurmountable sadness can be traced back to the initial (absent or intrusive?) bond with my mother. By talking, digging and deducing, we repeatedly conclude that there was no (genuine) attunement in my early years. My mother showered me with a kind of love that I couldn't receive because it didn't seem intended for me. She gives and gives abundantly, but she doesn't check what I need. For example, she lovingly prepares mussels with the best ingredients but doesn't consider that I've never liked mussels.

Through recounting my daily worries, we look for recurring patterns. We then place patterns within my relationship with my father, brother and mother. I often conclude that she wants to determine what I should or shouldn't do and what I should or shouldn't like. Bizarrely, she seems dominant on the one hand and wants to impose her will on me at all costs. On the other hand, she is dependent and seeks attention almost childishly, almost reversing the mother-daughter role. For example, I recently received far too much information from her about their sex life. She seems to endure dominant to painful sex but doesn't dare to object. On the contrary, she once advised me that 'If you let your spouse have their way, they will do everything you want afterwards'. Sex would make many things better in a relationship. And I knew there was much sex! My father found it a perfectly normal topic to bring up. There was a lot of ... well, let's say intimacy ... whether I wanted to hear it or not.

Even my virtually absent brother influences my view of sexuality. His statement that Disney and sex don't go together means that, to this day, I don't buy sleepwear with funny cartoons ... And he also mentions sex, but usually inappropriately, preferably using misogynistic statements. In my opinion, however, sex (or, more broadly, a relationship) should include love and tenderness, listening to each other and attuning to each other. Not imposing or humiliating ...

And that's where it clicks with my psychiatrist: he listens, checks, reasons and attunes ... He doesn't overwhelm me with his views or theories but tries to work with me on insight, acceptance and 'healing'. Sometimes, I also try to find answers in literature. Books about emotionally absent parents, parents who don't attune to what the child needs, read to me like diaries. I recognise myself so much in those stories. In their testimonies, I even read things I don't remember. I also discuss these things with my psychiatrist.

My now eighteen-month-long intense search is not yet over because I still encounter wrong thinking and acting patterns, sadness and loss that haven't been fully worked through and, therefore, haven't found a place. Too often, I'm overwhelmed by a lack, a pain I can't place.

The break-up with my ex highlights that this deficiency has always been present. My psychiatrist compares it to a child who only realises he was hungry when he got food. And I was hungry! Only now, in therapy, I realised I kept asking my boyfriend if he still loved me. I had and have such a need to check if I am good enough or if I am doing the right thing. Lack of self-confidence and self-love are a big issue for me. I feel like I exist only during my relationship with another significant person. I used to try so hard to make sure people saw me. (Please is my middle name.) After the break-up with my ex, I was suddenly completely alone. And that's how I still feel ... alone, without people around me who understand and see me. It's often said that I have everything to be happy, so I look for the cause – the fault – of my unhappiness in myself. Luckily, my psychiatrist points out that my 'problem' is not a luxury problem because even the princess on the pea doesn't sleep well in the end. So, I also learned that therapy doesn't consist of blaming myself but rather understanding myself. And so he keeps giving me, because I often ask for it (just like with my ex), a fatherly pat on the back that it's okay not to be OK yet. He guides me patiently, hand in hand, as it were. The feeling of not being alone, being understood and seen, and not being judged means a lot to me, as well as the confirmation that I'm doing well and raising the correct issues. Sometimes, I get into my car crying after a session and have to recover at home (sometimes with a glass of alcohol) from the released emotions and thoughts. And yet, I secretly look forward to my next session, curious about what else will surface. I attach great importance to the metaphors used to try to clarify what is so present yet invisible. I am progressing in small steps, gaining insights into my recurring 'wrong' patterns and, simultaneously, receiving support in breaking them. Therapy is changing my outlook on life, and I will emerge as a different person ... Now, I only hope that I may gradually experience what Charles Bukowski says so beautifully: 'I don't ask for happiness, just a little less pain.'

38 W.D.

I never thought I could tell my story after six years without shame, even with pride. I feel honoured to be able to do this. I especially want to inspire people and let them know you are never alone. Seeking help, and above all, allowing yourself to accept help, is the most important thing. That's how my journey began years ago. I was twenty-eight, in the prime of my life. I went out with friends, had the occasional boyfriend, and worked six days a week. I was on autopilot. Then the lights went out. I suddenly became emotionally unstable. I cried at the slightest thing and had no energy left. All I wanted to do was sleep. And preferably never wake up again.

Why I suddenly became unstable, in my opinion, is because I held myself together for too long, not considering the effect that traumas can have on your later years, how you stand in life and, above all, what kind of person you are in life. I had never considered what my upbringing and the relationship with my parents could leave behind. I ran away from my problems; I didn't want to be confronted with them. I waited too long to seek help, mainly out of ignorance. I found in my diary, written when I was twelve, that I needed a psychologist. Nobody ever read it. If I had received help then, my later years might have turned out differently, too.

Psychotherapy has strengthened me above all. I can now name, place and deal with my feelings more than ever. I'm cautiously learning to trust people again, and I'm not afraid to express my feelings. Through therapy, I've been given a second chance at life, and I'm grabbing it with both hands. I've become a better person for all the people around me, but especially for myself.

I had no experience with depression or mental health difficulties; I had never visited a psychiatrist or psychologist. So, I didn't immediately think I might have depression. My mum, who had herself been admitted to hospital and had suffered from depression, referred me to her psychiatrist. That's when I was told for the first time that I needed full admission. To begin with, twelve weeks. Words can't describe what went through my head. I was confused, sad and angry, but, above all, relieved somewhere deep in my heart that I was getting help and suddenly wasn't completely alone anymore. I was worried about my work but also had to let that go. Being unable to work for a long time was incredibly hard for me.

I had many friends and people around me who looked up to me; nobody was ever supposed to find out about this because I saw it as a weakness. I took the initiative myself to seek help and admission. What I've learned is that nobody can force you. You have to do it for yourself and by yourself. Minimising problems doesn't help; you have to acknowledge them. You must let them exist.

I had enormous difficulty trusting people. It took a long time before I could acclimatise to the new environment of the psychiatric ward. But I finally had peace. No stress, just time for myself. The therapy was complex but slowly started moving in the right direction. I had to talk about my feelings, something I had never done before. About my relationship with my parents. I didn't have an easy childhood, but I had never considered that I might have some trauma. Through music, expression and group therapy, I started digging, and a lot of sadness and anger came to the surface. All emotions that you can't cope with at first. I was supported both in a group and individually. I found it very difficult to speak in a group; I was usually silent during these sessions.

What I've learned above all is that you need to give it time and be kind to yourself. Allow yourself the time you need to heal because this is being ill and living with an emotional disability. I will never be cured; you must learn to live with this. In addition to my personality problems, I am susceptible and have obsessive-compulsive disorders (OCDs). Constantly living with obsessive thoughts is incredibly difficult. I'm usually very anxious, and sometimes I have panic attacks. What underlies my OCD is very delicate. I've had this since childhood, but then no help was offered. I had to learn to live with it on my own. Since becoming a mother, it has become much worse. The fear that my child might die preoccupies me every day. Every minute. That's why I have to perform specific actions every time with a positive thought to 'save' my child. Fear has the upper hand here, and it's challenging to fight against this day after day. I still struggle with this. I know it's related to separation anxiety. I'm afraid of losing my son and the real and close mother-child bond I have with him.

After my full admission, I was allowed a two-week trial discharge. It was only the beginning of a long road ahead. During this phase, I restored contact with a lost great love. This was the solution to all my problems. We moved in together, and I became pregnant. Only I didn't know that he would leave me for another woman after five months. I didn't think I would become a single mother with many more obstacles. Only the love for my child pulled me through. I wasn't aware at the time that this was a repetition of a toxic relationship. I've never known spontaneous love; I always had to beg for it. The complicated relationship I had with my father manifested itself years later in my choice of partner. I never had a stable father figure, which made my relationships with men difficult.

In my early years, I was mainly raised by my grandparents. My father had a relationship with a prostitute and had a drug addiction. It was the opposite world; I had to be the parent figure. I had to grow up very quickly. I also have a complicated love-hate relationship with my mother. She had to take on both roles because I didn't have a father figure. And she couldn't cope with that. My mum also had mental health problems and an addiction. She was also admitted to the hospital. Every story and every journey are different; I didn't take the same path as her.

In the meantime, through therapy, I've found a way to forgive my mother. Because ultimately, I do love her. I tried to realise that she did everything she could but didn't know anything better. If she had sought help earlier, she might have become a different and better person. I'm fortunate that I started therapy at a young age. This is also what has made me the person I am today. I try to do better as a mother than I ever knew. I'm very conscious of my child's upbringing. However, I also must realise that a perfect mother and upbringing don't exist.

I can say that my pregnancy wasn't planned, but it did save my life. The arrival of my child gave me a reason to live again, a primal instinct that emerged. I had never felt this before. I had to live to care for my child. Suicide was no longer an option. The word suicide. A word I had never been able to write before but which occupied me every day.

I don't believe in fate or that things happen for a reason. This is an excuse that people use. Things happen because people make a choice. You are responsible for the choices you make, whether consciously or unconsciously. I had unconsciously chosen the wrong man for the umpteenth time – the father of my child. Don't get me wrong, if I wanted a child with anyone, it was with him. So I'll never regret this. He was the greatest love I've ever known, but unfortunately, the wrong one. I needed support and understanding, someone who would stand by me. But he couldn't give me that, and we grew apart. I didn't lose him; I outgrew him.

After the birth of my son, I stayed away from the psychiatric ward for a while. I then decided to continue my therapy. I felt I wasn't finished yet. The break-up with my ex-partner and the beginning of life as a single mother allowed me to start my psychotherapeutic process. I was personally supported by my personal nurse, individually and in a group, by the psychiatrist and the psychotherapist. I got a lot out of the energy and the stories you share with fellow patients.

Everyone has their problems and stories. The support you get from each other and the emotional bonds you create all contribute to your healing process. I quickly realised this wasn't fleeting; it required time and attention. And above all, patience. Patience with yourself and the path you have to take to get better. I started intensive day therapy again. Full admission was no longer necessary. These were my working days. I am working on myself to be a better person and to be able to live with my shortcomings.

I then moved back in with my mum and my five-month-old son. I had no money or furniture to afford a roof over my head again. I had to start from scratch. The psychiatric ward was my haven. A healing process is something with many ups and downs. When you think you've hit rock bottom and can't sink more profoundly, you go up again. Small euphorias and minor setbacks.

I could express my emotions again through music therapy and playing the piano. Through expression, I dared to think further than my head sometimes allowed. Through psychotherapy, I learned to trust people and to speak in groups. Through individual support, I felt again that I wasn't alone. Months went by until I was stable enough to reduce my therapy to half-day sessions and then further reduce it to a few sessions per week, which is called aftercare.

A healing process works in stages; you can't run if you can't walk yet. During this period, I had the time and space to seek further help finding a house and gradually save some money again to buy furniture. I sometimes can't believe how far I've come as I write this. Occasionally, I must be reminded that I can be proud of this.

I found it very difficult to say goodbye to the psychiatric ward, but I had to let go of that, too. I had to spread my wings and learn to fly alone now. I still go to see my psychiatrist for consultations every few weeks and my psychologist about once a week.

At the moment, I'm in a good place in life. I'm progressively working as a beautician, which has always been my passion but which I lost for a while and couldn't find anymore. I have my own house, which I've made my home with heart and soul. I have my son and have recently been in a budding relationship. I've also built some savings, so I'm no longer financially dependent on anyone. I owe all this to those who believed in me and helped me find myself again. But especially to myself. Because I was the only person who could make a change.

I've lost many people who didn't understand this; that's just part of it. Not everyone thinks mental health is a priority. Some people think you're crazy once they know you're going to a psychiatrist. At the same time, it's just about an emotional deficit. Not everyone is lucky enough to be born with a silver spoon in their mouth. Nobody chooses their parents or family. But what you do choose is your happiness.

I can still have bad days and be brought down by a particular memory. But I'm not depressed anymore. I'm cured of my depression, but I will always struggle with a kind of emotional disability. I'm working on my procrastination and still learning every day. I'm learning to be happy by living alone and making the most of the little things. I appreciate what I have instead of what I've lost. I didn't know how strong I was until I saw my son's eyes and saw myself. I've learned to draw strength from things I didn't know existed. The more you find yourself, the more life will find you.

I've broken off contact with my father for several years now after the death of my grandmother. I've come to terms with her loss (she was like a mother to me). I miss her every day. My relationship with my mum has never been better than it is now. We recently received the terrible news that she has cancer and that it has spread. I want to make the most of the time we have left in all the love we can feel. Because if she's not there anymore, I'll be an orphan. Then I will not only figuratively have no parents anymore but also literally.

I want to inspire people with my story and tell them you are never alone. That life can be beautiful, depending on how you look at it. For me, happiness lies in small things. He who does not honour the small does not deserve the great. I'm happy with a cup of coffee, the sun shining, my son's laughter, and being able to buy food and cook nice meals. My darkest moments have led me to success. I used to be led around; now it feels like I'm in charge. I want the life I'm entitled to; I put myself first in life, along with my little son.

Chapter 4

Finishing Touches

1 The Typical Journey

After their testimony was written down and sent, almost all patients discussed their text with me again. This was an excellent opportunity to highlight certain matters, to elaborate on points, or to provide additional questions, considerations or comments. For some, it was an arduous process, but everyone found it educational in one way or another. You don't look back on your psychotherapy from a helicopter perspective every day. You get to explicitly articulate things on paper/in black and white even less often. In these concluding remarks, I evidently refrain from personal interpretation and limit myself to generalisations. First, I will discuss what psychotherapy roughly means for both parties. Then, I will discuss the assumptions or presumptions regarding what a psychoanalytic form of psychotherapy would lead to.

Initially, most patients highly value their psychotherapy. They are listened to attentively and treated delicately and tactfully by someone who makes every effort to understand them quickly and as well as possible. Psychotherapy even has something alluring about it because the patient is invited to say everything to a receptive and non-judgemental figure. Many patients welcome this opportunity to unburden themselves, like confessing something and experiencing the relief of absolution.

But something else, more profound, is also at play. Our mother was in a state of grace during our first months, so if all goes well, she was exceptionally well equipped to meet our biological and psychological needs. This is called the primary maternal preoccupation by psychoanalyst Donald Winnicott and the motherhood constellation by infant researcher Daniel Stern. The land of milk and honey is where the luckiest among us are born. We have fallen, like Obelix, into a vat of magic potion and derive strength and (self-) confidence from this foundation. Psychotherapy, in many respects, also begins with such a honeymoon period. The psychotherapist has an open mind and focuses on the patient's contribution. They bring all their knowledge and skill to bear in order to understand the patient's problem as well as possible, ultimately making it even their 'job'. I dare to suggest, somewhat provocatively, that it

DOI: 10.4324/9781003528067-4

often happens that psychotherapy is prematurely terminated (by the patient) or perhaps even stopped (by the therapist), namely before or when this honeymoon period ends.

As psychotherapy progresses (or rather, truly begins), the patient starts to tell more and more things that they do not understand or were not initially intending to speak about. Pleasure begins to give way again to the kind of burden that had led them to therapy. Guilty or shameful secrets and fantasies bubble up. They provoke, for example, fear of punishment or retribution, loss of self-worth or the esteem of others. During this phase, the patient begins to experience more mixed feelings towards the undertaking or the psychotherapist.

On the one hand, they want to continue their self-examination; on the other hand, they want to return to earlier ways of 'adaptation' that they had developed for themselves in a more or less satisfactory way. They get into a dilemma. They must choose between the devil and the deep blue sea: the familiar psychological discomforts of their earlier life or the seemingly dangerous and, therefore, unknown possibilities that open up before them.

Sometimes, in the meantime – without realising it – they have reached a point of no return. For example, they have become attached to their therapist. Or they may become convinced that their psychotherapist 'knows'. The patient may still – often haphazardly, but also if they don't know what they want to get away from – see that they are taking a 'flight'. If they stop their psychotherapy, the lingering feeling that a task begun has remained unfinished will continue to haunt them to a greater or lesser extent. A psychotherapeutic process can, therefore, proceed in one piece and, as it were, 'in instalments'. Regarding emotional costs and benefits, the patient has broken off contact at a certain point when a new equilibrium seems to have been reached regarding costs and benefits. They have dropped the thread but later pick it up again – whether or not it is a result of life events that trigger something or after necessary or unnecessary wanderings.

Suffering is an essential motive for seeking help and an engine of the psychotherapeutic process. Whenever the patient believes they have found a *modus vivendi*, this engine starts to sputter. In addition, however, there is also the desire to understand themselves better. Call it a form of curiosity about their internal affairs that has motivated the patient to seek psychotherapy or with which they are, as it were, infected by their psychotherapist. They then identify to some extent with the desire of the psychoanalytic therapist and want to know the details of what their unconscious has to say about their joys and sorrows.

2 The Psychoanalytic Experience: A Concave Approach

The psychoanalytic psychotherapist adopts a concave posture at the beginning of the psychotherapy and each session. They try to register and receive with their 'satellite dish'. They pay attention to mental contents and how the patient processes and expresses them. They help to investigate and metabolise. Not least, they are looking for subliminal clues and are particularly interested in context and subtext.

Sooner or later, the psychotherapist becomes essential to the patient: a key figure. The most unmistakable sign is when the psychotherapist begins to feature in the patient's dreams or nightmares. The story then unfolds more and more within the consulting room. It takes place there. It becomes a unique opportunity to learn first-hand what or who the patient's history revolves around and try to give it a different direction or outcome.

It is a serious undertaking, but it also has a play-like quality. The therapist is not only a listener or observer but also a participant. They want to understand what is going on in their patient's head and heart and build a relationship with the patient that offers sufficient safety and trust within professional boundaries. They take into account the needs and tendencies of the patient, which they simultaneously explore and help to articulate as they shift and develop. The patient can learn a lot about themselves from this. But so can the psychotherapist. Perfect parents exist, but they don't have kids. If parents cannot acknowledge their shortcomings, the child has to pay the price. The same applies to psychotherapists and their patients.

The psychotherapist's method in all this is scientific and empirical. They form hypotheses that can explain surface phenomena, and, through (trial) interpretations, they try to test these hypotheses. Confirmation or denial by the patient is not taken at face value. The former may, for example, indicate compliance, the latter resistance to authority. Instead, what is assessed is whether the 'material' (the data) that the patient produces following the interpretation confirms, refines or refutes the hypothesis is assessed. Psychoanalysis is, of course, primarily the science of the particular. What specific and unique laws govern and restrict the patient's experience? Paradoxically, psychoanalysis is a science of unreason.

Psychoanalytic treatment necessarily involves a degree of regression. This happens thanks to free association and the non-critical and non-intrusive presence of the analyst in a setting characterised by introspection and understanding. The patient, so to speak, becomes somewhat more childish. They return to more primitive ways of feeling and behaving and to a more egocentric preoccupation. while at the same time becoming more dependent on the analyst. In this way, a second-chance upbringing occurs with a benevolent therapist who contributes to recollecting, understanding and processing past experiences in an atmosphere of positive acceptance.

Clinical psychotherapy, in particular, can be life-saving in many cases, but it can also involve a long and profound operation. Sometimes, the analogy with surgical intervention applies, accompanied by a period of intensive care, significant dependence (such as temporarily supporting or taking over vital functions) and bed rest. A patient who is still mobile and walking before hospitalisation may require a long rehabilitation or convalescence post-operatively.

3 The Past in the Present: Unveiling Repetition

A concise description of psychoanalysis comes from Horacio Etchegoyen, former president of the International Psychoanalytical Association. In his standard work on the fundamentals of psychoanalytic technique, he calls psychoanalysis a method that recognises the past in the present and distinguishes it through interpretation. One of the most compelling aspects of psychoanalytic psychotherapy is indeed the opportunity it provides to be able to remove the spectacles of our fantasy and our past. This is done by examining how patients view and approach their environment, particularly the therapist.

To some extent, the patient can tell their story, but, at least equally, this history manifests in how they move within the consulting room and relate to the psychotherapist. The latter must be able to tolerate the patient making all sorts of things of them. They must also facilitate the expression of all their feelings (even those that are least refined or most intense). They must be prepared to be loved, idealised and desired but also to be avoided, mocked, envied or criticised. In the meantime, they must maintain their equanimity and observational, verbalising and insightful abilities. They move, as it were, between emotional developmental support and interpretative microsurgery.

'What is repeated must be remembered' is one of the classic psychoanalytic principles. Whoever does not know their past is doomed to repeat it. Our problems do not come out of the blue but are connected with what we have made of our history. Mentally, in psychotherapy, we retrace our steps with the patient. Where and why did I end up in a particular street? How far has this taken me away from the path I might have been able to or wanted to take? In which direction do I need to adjust to get 'there' to the extent that is possible?

4 Addressing Neuroses: The Oedipus Complex

The original psychoanalytic domain is that of so-called neuroses. These are problems that we are at odds with or that are entangled in internal affairs, which evidently complicates our foreign affairs. They often find their roots in and during our early childhood years. Initially, our mouth is central. We take in what tastes good and spit out what tastes terrible. We oscillate between heaven and hell. It's a matter of being hungry or satiated, fulfilled or in dire straits. Subsequently, the tone of our relationship with autonomy, power and control is set. Toddlers are the terrible twos. A duo turns into a duel. Who's the boss? Whose will prevails? Finally, the sexual comes to the forefront; we experienced first crushes on figures from our immediate environment and would seemingly have gone to any lengths for exclusivity.

Which child doesn't want to be bigger and/or older? Which child doesn't want to marry mum or dad? Or which child doesn't want to *be* mum or dad? Initially, the child needs to be lovingly 'placed' within a complex network of relationships of which it is not the centre. If all goes well, this intervention is a lever for two developmental tasks: separating and leading one's life and building or acquiring a (gender) identity.

The reader understands that, in plain language, I'm referring to the famous Oedipus complex. According to Freud, it's the core complex of neuroses and, for many of the therapeutic processes in neurosis, this complex turns out to be both the culmination and the *pièce de résistance* (main course and point of most outstanding resistance). In a nutshell, the Oedipus complex regulates who 'enjoys' whom and what. A third party forbids the parent from the child and the child from the parent. Thus, a forbidden and impossible (because incestuous) 'something' is placed under the law. Law and desire henceforth become two sides of the same coin. However, the law or prohibition implicitly and inevitably evokes its transgression.

Neurotic patients struggle with ambivalent feelings, are grappling with sexual and/or aggressive and/or narcissistic tendencies, and in various ways ward off all kinds of guilt-ridden, shameful or generally frightening content. They are often involved in hidden or covert triangular relationships, and variations on the theme mean the saying 'two is company, three is a crowd' applies to them. This leads, in the form of the disguised return of the repressed, to problems/symptoms of all kinds. They are complex and full of knots and twists; therefore, they barely see the wood for the trees. The psychotherapeutic task is to cut the crap. It's about searching for underlying patterns that repeat themselves in variations on a theme, and it often takes a lot of time and effort to get them out of their system.

5 Beyond Neurosis: More Fundamental Problems

Most (mainly British) post-Freudians have moved to other borderlands of mental health problems. This concerns a domain where more fundamental difficulties exist regarding basic trust, stability or constancy, and symbolising capacity. They are situated in a more archaic register where and when unbearable emotional content is cast off rather than banished or repressed to an inner foreign country. Here, forms of psychoanalytic therapy with a broader scope are imposed based on an adapted theory. Jacques Lacan and Heinz Kohut remain distinct figures: Lacan, with his so-called return to the early Freud, who read dreams, slips of the tongue, symptoms (and even the unconscious in general) primarily as a text; and Kohut, who – by absolutising his self-psychology – has distanced himself from North American psychoanalysis.

Classically, the psychoanalytic process was characterised by deconstruction. A proliferation of layers of meaning formed over time in the person and around the symptom is dismantled. In this way, an attempt is made to return to their core or root and to take other paths. Gradually, however, psychoanalysis has also taken a more constructive turn. Something is added to the material the patient brings. Freud distinguished between sculptor and painter. The former takes something away; the image is in the wood or marble but must be brought to light. The latter adds something to the canvas; it is coated with – often multiple – layers of paint and brushstrokes.

I refer first, regarding the transition to these more constructive developments, to the work of Melanie Klein, who worked intensively with severely disturbed children using play therapy and thus entered and highlighted primitive layers from the earliest mother-child relationship; to Donald Winnicott, who, as a paediatrician, saw thousands of mothers and babies in his practice and distilled original ideas about the use of the psychotherapist as a developmental object; and finally to Wilfred Bion, who worked with groups of military and psychotic patients and conceived of the potentially transformative function of the mother/psychotherapist.

Interestingly, contemporary neuroscientific research (for example, by Allan Schore) also shows much preverbal communication in early life, namely between both right hemispheres of the brain, where feelings, experiences and impressions are primarily processed. This contributes to affect regulation and to the construction of the self. Thus, psychoanalysis can also be a shared emotional experience from which the symbolism of language and thought can still be born in a kind of joint (ad)venture.

6 Technical Metaphors

In Freud's complete oeuvre, his technical writings occupy a minimal space regarding the number of pages. However, they largely retain their importance to this day. In the 'Setting the Stage' section, I already referred to concepts such as transference, resistance and free association by the patient, and free-floating attention by the psychotherapist. To avoid jargon, I can further compare the psychoanalytic process to some household activities. Thus, the psychotherapist is something like a vacuum cleaner. His silence is an action that can have as much effect as a motor action. The best way to get someone to talk is to be silent yourself. In this way, material is sucked up, even from under the carpet.

Instead of interpretation, I propose the tin-opener (Dutch *blikopener* = eye-opener). The cracks or crevices in (the tin cans of) speech provide insight into previously closed-off content, even when their expiry date has passed and toxic gases are starting or threatening to escape. With this simple tool, we can open or widen the tin. In this way, we can notice things that repeat themselves, and the memory of their roots can be an excellent antidote.

Finally, I find the metaphor of the iron helpful. Various creases and (true or false) folds have formed in us over time. It is a matter of investigating which folds and from where, from whom or when they came. To get them out of our system, as anyone who irons knows, we must repeatedly go over them in various ways and from different angles.

Contrary to what mainly inexperienced therapists think, a single interpretation does not bring about change. Resistance persists, even after the most accurate interpretation. Working through is necessary. Habits are formed but also disappear only after sufficient repetition. In one of his technical writings, Freud emphasises – besides repetition and remembrance – the importance of working through. Integration of interpretations into the personality becomes possible only by becoming aware, in a lived-through way, of specific patterns that repeat themselves in variations on the theme and in different circumstances (also within the psychotherapeutic encounter itself).

It is precisely in this working through that psychoanalysis distinguishes itself from many other forms of psychotherapy. Through all this, old automatisms can be replaced, with trial and error and with varying success, by more updated ones. It is the longest and, in a sense, also the most discouraging phase in any psychotherapy. The patient knows what patterns he has become entangled in; he also sees how it could have come to this. Yet he continues to stumble over the same stones, causing him to want to throw in the towel on that miserable psychotherapeutic undertaking (if not his life).

It is beyond the scope of this book to delve into further technical details. Still, I will explain what kinds of developments psychoanalytic therapies are supposed to lead to so that the reader can test the testimonies against this.

7 Freud's Aims: Towards Greater Freedom

Of course, the primary aim is to make the patient more aware of unconscious contents and processes. Initially, they feel unwell and do not understand what's wrong. We then work together to explore recurring patterns in their life. We often use, so to speak, the rule of three. We can all miss things or make mistakes – *errare humanum est*. To err is human. The second part of this Seneca quote is less often remembered: *perseverare diabolicum*. To persist in error is diabolical.

For Freud, this diabolical element resides in the demonic nature of the unconscious. We are internally possessed by drives and other forces, sometimes even caricatured figures. Psychoanalysis is the science of traces. Tracing and highlighting repetitions invites the patient to discover deeper layers through these cracks. Layer by layer, we reach older findings around which ever-changing derivatives have formed over time.

In the classical Freudian view, the patient doesn't become better and wiser but somewhat sadder and wiser through this undertaking. During a psychotherapeutic process, the neurotic patient, in particular, can lose many illusions about others, the world and themselves. Our Dutch colleague Antonie Ladan succinctly calls the psychoanalyst a 'disillusionist'. More positively formulated, we become more realistic. If things went well, our parents made great efforts to make us believe in fairy tales and Santa Claus. Ideally, they also instilled faith and trust in us in other ways. We all need dreams and fantasies to retreat into our world occasionally and keep the ever-advancing armies of reality at bay. But we must also be able to leave fairyland behind in good time to achieve things.

The pleasure principle, where we want everything immediately, must give way to the reality principle, of which science, according to Freud, is indeed the epitome. We must, especially in psychotherapy, be able to postpone instant gratification and first bite into the sour apples before being able to savour various fruits with an even greater appetite.

We have a large assortment of defence mechanisms, and thankfully so. Without them, life would be unbearable at times, if not impossible. However, the aim is to expand rigid, stereotypical or counterproductive defence mechanisms flexibly and variably into the broadest possible repertoire. Humour is one of the highest. It allows the expression of scabrous or malicious content in such a way that it evokes pleasure for both the individual and their environment. It is one of the most common forms of sublimation, where drives find satisfaction both pro-socially and without repression.

Freud may be deterministic and seek underlying reasons or causes for every phenomenon (even the most banal), yet his psychoanalysis aims for greater freedom. It's not about negative freedom, à la Isaiah Berlin, but positive freedom. English has different words for this. There's liberty, freedom from external or superior constraints, and freedom to lead one's own life according to one's own will and autonomously (Greek: *nomos* = law). The psychoanalytic project is dedicated to positive freedom. It has an emancipatory quality, as it aims to liberate the patient from a harness of symptoms, inhibitions and anxieties or – underlying these – from fixed patterns that hinder freedom.

Freud's model was initially a bio-psycho-social drive-defence model. There is a conflict between lower and higher forces. Upbringing and civilisation tame or temper drives, but we pay a price for this. The struggle between wild impulsiveness (the id) and the dos and don'ts of the micro- and macro-culture in which the child grows up (the superego) rages internally and is never fully resolved.

After he introduces narcissism, the conflict seems to shift to that between self-love and love for another. Do we ever become sufficiently self-aware? How do we evolve to a form of love where the other is recognised and loved in their alterity? Freud prefers the contrast between illness and health over good and evil and doesn't develop this new avenue much further. However, another conflict develops in his thinking, namely between the life and death drives. The former leads to bonding and disintegration, which he also links to love and hate. Although he systematically integrates these two drives into his thinking from their introduction, they only receive their fullest elaboration with Melanie Klein and Jacques Lacan, each in their own specific way.

Freud is an evolutionary thinker, and psychoanalysis aims to restart or get a stalled or skewed development back on track. Progression must gain the upper hand over fixation and regression. It also aims to bring our mental apparatus (the ego, as Freud calls it) to optimal development. The ability to tolerate anxiety and frustration, the constructive use of defence mechanisms, and our reality testing are all signs of increased ego strength. Contemporary theories about attachment in mutual connection with mentalising ability connect with what Freud called the ego or self-preservation drives. Especially at the beginning of his thinking, they were clearly distinguished from (in the broadest sense of the word) sexual drives.

Freud was, in a sense, also a rationalist. *Wo Es war, soll Ich werden.* The ego (the steering wheel) must take over where the id was. Incidentally, the superego can also be cruel and primitive and needs to be mitigated by analysis. True morality is not a matter of an eye for an eye, a tooth for a tooth, but rather a matter of breast for breast. The love of and for this good object constitutes the core of the conscience. Not the fear of a pursuing or sadistic executioner nor the socially constructed norms and values of an inner tyrant.

8 From Patriarchy to Matriarchy: (Post-) Kleinian Perspectives

It is now appropriate to bridge the gap to the design of psychoanalysis in the view of later 'greats', starting with Melanie Klein. Fundamentally, for her, our psychic life revolves around the mother/breast (as a fountain of milk but also of warmth, love, security and understanding). While Freud was phallocentric and focused on the time of the patriarchy, Klein delves into the matriarchy that precedes it in our (cultural and personal) history.

The first order we bring to chaos from a young age is between white and black, day and night, the presence or absence of mama or the mother (breast). The absence of the safe good is initially perceived as a threatening evil in our inner and outer world. Both worlds are equally imbued with animism: they become populated with fairy-tale or ghostly representations. It is still a magical universe. In this phase, the good must be kept safe from the evil, and representations of others or ourselves are initially split. In the child's mind (like in fairy tales) caricatured and two-dimensional figures predominate. They embody a clear dividing line between good and evil, fairy and hag, lovely and malicious.

Only in a later phase do alloys of good and evil come about, and evil is also located more within than outside ourselves. Our anxieties change shape. They evolve from paranoid or persecutory anxieties to depressive anxieties. We then worry about the evil we inflict on others (instead of vice versa), and we try to repair our misdeeds with good deeds and thus repair the damage. We also get a more realistic and nuanced picture of others and ourselves. As adults, we oscillate between what Klein calls a schizoid-paranoid and a depressive position.

Especially when we are in trouble, the former often takes over again. However, in an optimal course of events, the depressive position prevails. Realism precedes magical thinking; evil is not first externalised and then fought as a (more or less natural) enemy. We remain sufficiently aware of our share, taking responsibility for our mistakes or failures, even when we have sinned unconsciously or unintentionally.

However, both positions can be helpful because black-and-white thinking regarding these positions needs to be transcended. For example, we would not know the idealisation of infatuation without the schizoid-paranoid position. The villains of this world must also be recognised as such if we are to combat or neutralise them effectively. The fact that Hitler loved painting and was fond of his dog does not change the fact that he had to be eliminated. In other words, splitting can be advantageous or adaptive. Conversely, ambivalence can be paralysing. 'On the one hand, this, on the other hand', can lead to endless doubts or indecisiveness that make any decisive action impossible.

Our ego and superego develop in parallel. There is a difference between mercilessly beating yourself up out of guilt and trying to make amends for the evil you have caused. The former is a primitive conscience in full action. It is (in this case mainly self-) destructive. Only the second, more mature form of conscience function serves a constructive, namely reparative, purpose.

Another Kleinian opposition is that between envy and gratitude. It is possible that the other (or breast) is not attacked or destroyed because it is terrible but because it is good. The good is envied and, therefore, cannot be incorporated as good into our inner world. It is a highly destructive phenomenon, which Klein links to the death drive. However, not all envy is destructive. As in the film *I, Tonya*, you can injure your competing figure skater and thus eliminate or destroy her. Still, you can also develop yourself to surpass or equal your idols. This was once called (Latin) *aemulatio*: noble rivalry.

Finally, Kleinian psychoanalysis attributes great importance to developing our symbolising capacity. Many children and patients cannot yet express themselves very well. They need a mother or psychotherapist who 'feeds' them with images and words with which they can illuminate or brighten their inner world. Expressing our mental content this way has both pro-social and beneficial consequences for our well-being. Symbolising ability underlies play and creativity. Being able to grasp various impressions or experiences not literally but figuratively significantly increases both one's own and others' freedom of movement.

In the wake of Klein, Wilfred Bion developed a theory about (the development of) our thinking. Thinking here must be distinguished from (purely) rational thinking. According to Bion, we need truth as much as we need oxygen. Only we cannot breathe it in its pure form. Our mind must evolve to increase our mental capacity for sensations and emotions. If not, we try to eliminate them in all possible and impossible ways. Mutely.

Besides 'L' for love and 'H' for hate, he introduces 'K' for knowledge (although knowledge is more related to *savoir* than to *connaître*) as a vector that determines our psychic life. The psychoanalytic process moves in the direction of L and K. In the second half of his theorising, he also introduces 'O'. It is the ultimately unknown, but also unknowable and nameless being with which we must come into sufficient contact to deal with the things of life in a more personal and original way.

9 From One-Person to Two-Person Psychology: Relational Approaches

While Melanie Klein focused primarily on the intrapsychic aspects of our unconscious fantasies, in Bion's psychoanalytic undertaking, communication takes on a more significant role. Between baby and mother and between patient and psychotherapist, a kind of mental coitus occurs from which thought is born.

At a more profound and earlier level, much communication takes place non-verbally. The baby/patient, for example, may bombard the mother/psychotherapist with incomprehensible or unbearable mental contents. They are, as it were, dumped or downloaded and take possession of the receiver's mind. In this way, the 'sender' may attempt to communicate something without words or, by evacuating these contents, try to avoid the pain of thinking. Ideally, the mother/psychotherapist does not reject or reflect these contents. Instead, the mental contents evoked are recognised, detoxified and translated. They are returned to be better digested and incorporated into the developing psyche of the baby/patient.

In more technical terms, Bion speaks of raw or traumatic experiences, which he calls beta-elements. The reverie or alpha function of the mother/psychotherapist must mediate these. Through playful interaction, she alphabetises us more, or less. In this context, I quote a *bon mot* from child psychotherapist Gaston Cluckers: *Elle pense, donc je suis.* I translate: If (and only if) the mother thinks, can (the) I be.

Over time, psychoanalysis has indeed evolved from a one-person to two-person psychology and from an intrapsychic to a more interpersonal focus. Alongside Wilfred Bion, Donald Winnicott is largely responsible for this. Unlike Sigmund Freud, Melanie Klein and Jacques Lacan, he is an unsystematic thinker. He has a more poetic than scientific approach and develops pieces of theory from $n = 1$.

On the one hand, he situates himself within the post-Kleinian line. For example, what he calls the 'capacity for concern' is simply another name for Klein's depressive position. Initially, the child experiences a ruthless phase and is only concerned with itself and not yet with the other. Only in a later phase, namely with sufficient psychological maturation, is the mental state of the other also taken into account. This is accompanied by the evolution from subjective to objective objects: figures are initially seen as an extension or variant of oneself, and only later are they recognised in their radical otherness, with their feelings and sensitivities.

The transition from so-called narcissistic- to object-love takes place in a transitional or intermediate space. This is arguably Winnicott's most significant contribution to psychoanalysis, and he is the most frequently cited of all its authors. In the coming and going of the mother, particular objects emerge, which Winnicott calls transitional objects. They arise in the play of sound and light between mother and child who engage together in play (Latin: *in lusio*).

These are animate objects that, in a sense, contain the body (not of Christ but) of the mother. The inseparable blanket, comforter or cuddly toy is highly precious and irreplaceable and comes from both inside and outside. It is a co-creation between baby and mother, poet and muse, patient and psychotherapist. It is the relic of moments of encounter where both touch each other (to express it somewhat sublimely), like on the ceiling of the Sistine Chapel.

A reasonable interpretation can then have something of this transitional object. Within the session, it even shows some formal resemblance to a work of art. It is unsaturated so that the patient can still add all kinds of additional meaning to it. It embraces the allusion (Latin.: *ad lusio*), which gives the patient the freedom to find themselves in it, or not, to a greater or lesser extent. It is the fruit of both partners' (also unconscious) psyche. Finally, a *colloque singulier* acquires its meaning within their unique encounters, based on which a shared history and idiom develop. At the same time, and precisely for all these reasons, it is difficult for third parties or outsiders to follow. Therefore, unlike a work of art, it cannot claim universal validity.

The transitional space within which these objects or phenomena occur is the space of play. It is an interface between fantasy and reality and between inside and outside. Both belief and disbelief are suspended. Compare it to a cinema film. You must forget that it is merely projecting moving images onto a screen. You have to believe in it. But you must also remember that it is only a projection and that the characters, for example, are not shot dead. So you also shouldn't believe in it. Over time, the transitional space will extend to the most diverse cultural expressions.

Winnicott compares psychotherapy to two people playing together. The ability to play is closely linked to several other skills. Thus, he distinguishes between the true and the false self. The true self can lose itself in play. To surrender (not to disintegration but) to non-integration. It does not have to hold itself together. It has sufficient security to let itself go into play. Defence is unnecessary. It can simply *be* without having to *do* anything. It can be alone, but it can also only *be*. It has experienced a sufficiently safe mothering environment that does not leave the child to its fate but also leaves it alone.

Winnicott conceived the psychoanalytic setting as a corrective or reparative mother-child relationship in which the psychotherapist offers maternal functions that were lacking or disturbed in the original dyad. The psychotherapist becomes a new (developmental) object and a secure base. The experience of a maternal presence that is not intrusive but reliable and highly attuned to the patient's inner world creates a transformative experience within the psychoanalytic encounter. According to the British psychoanalyst Christopher Bollas, this would produce an existential rather than a representational knowing because it cannot be said, only experienced.

10 The Self: Kohutian Contributions

Besides the post-Kleinian and relational approaches that Winnicott respectively follows and opens up, Winnicott also emphasises the self for the first time. This latter perspective is taken up by Heinz Kohut and absolutised by him into a fundamental psychoanalytic framework. To avoid pejorative connotations, Kohut calls all narcissistic disorders self-disorders and develops his self-psychology.

He will understand psychological problems almost exclusively as difficulties that people experience with their sense of self, self-love, self-image, self-esteem, and so on. The other (in other words, the object, starting with the mother) fulfils self-object functions, that is, functions in the service of the self. The child/patient needs sufficient empathic mirroring to develop a positive and stable self-image. The child/patient also needs to idealise the parent/psychotherapist and derive his sense of self and self-esteem from it.

When this self-object function fails or is deficient for whatever reason, not disintegration (of the ego) but fragmentation (of the self) occurs. There is disorientation and shame. Kohut reads various symptomatic behaviours (sexual, aggressive, perverse, or toxic) as the product of such fragmentation. Sufficient empathic mirroring is then necessary to process narcissistic injury. Under a regime of optimal frustration and in a back-and-forth of injury and recovery, the self gains strength.

I mention this (in my opinion, less critical and specifically psychoanalytic) school of thought because it can be imperative in building and maintaining a therapeutic relationship. Not least because the psychotherapist – when there is a bump in the road – tries to ascertain where and how he has fallen short in his self-object function and how the patient (re)acts to this 'catastrophe'.

11 Lacanian Insights: The Imaginary, Symbolic and Real

Jacques Lacan is the most distinctive of the post-Freudians (also regarding the finality of the psychoanalytic process). Although I explicitly am not a Lacanian, I nonetheless count him among the most important alongside Freud because of the breadth (clinical, philosophical-anthropological, and general cultural) of his thought. He distances himself from the emphasis placed after Freud – particularly in North America – on the ego and that placed by the British on the imaginary. Instead, he sees the ego as a (literal) *trompe l'oeil* or a blind spot. We identify with a (mirror) image that does not correspond with our self and thus alienates us from ourselves.

Let's clarify that this controversy surrounding the ego is essentially a semantic issue. What, after all, is meant by the term ego? Classically Freudian, the ego concerns an intrapsychic instance, a cockpit from which the plane is steered. Lacan conceives of it primarily as specular. It is an imaginary formation that gives us an illusion of wholeness and mastery, which he considers fake and fictitious. Although Lacan was firmly rooted in French psychiatry and initially focused primarily on psychosis, a large part of the Parisian *beau monde* or intelligentsia attended his famous seminars and/or ended up on his couch. It is, therefore, no wonder that, over time, his practice came to be dominated by patients with an intellectualising style and narcissistic and/or neurotic problems.

For Lacan, the psychoanalytic process aims not so much to liberate our ego but to liberate us *from* it. Not least by letting the subject of our unconscious/ the unconscious subject speak. This is the subject that only appears in the speech act. It is not the subject of what is said but the subject of the saying. The word 'I' with which a sentence begins never (entirely) coincides with the one who produces the words. The subject – to which Lacan gives precedence over the ego – only finds expression in moments of full speech.

For Lacan, what is essential is that humankind, as a speaking being or as a linguistic animal, is marked by the law of symbolic language and the symbolic order that irrevocably separates us from ourselves. We are symbolising and meaning-giving beings. We share the imaginary order to some extent with animals, but only this latter symbolic register is specifically human and separates us from (our) nature. We yearn (back) for immediacy (with Mother/ nature), but when we transgress the laws of the symbolic order to achieve this, we end up in an unpleasant or destructive wasteland.

Although he denies its influence, Lacan is an existentialist like Jean-Paul Sartre. For this French philosopher, things were '*(plein-d')être*', full of being. Humankind, on the other hand, is a lack-of-being, a want-to-be or '*néant*'. In things, essence precedes existence, while in humanity, conversely, the essence is only derived from existence. Humankind is condemned to the freedom of making something of themselves. Even though they often act in bad faith and hide behind a conventional form of being. Everyone's life is the sum of (conscious and unconscious) choices, and humans essentially bring about themselves and their world.

From the moment we learn to speak, we do not cease to (de)scribe ourselves. But something also persists that does not let itself be written. After the Lacan of the Imaginary and the Symbolic, the later Lacan primarily foregrounds the Real. It is the part of the Thing (German: *Ding an sich*) that cannot be imagined or expressed: unknown and unknowable. The Real, by definition, cannot be spoken, yet most Lacanians count drive and trauma as belonging to this register, for example. It also ensures that we are never (entirely) finished talking because, ultimately, images and words fatally fall short.

Freud already spoke of the mycelium or the navel of the dream. Even after analysis, the dream retains an opaque, unanalysable core. In connection with the symptom, Freud speaks of the mother-of-pearl that the oyster forms around a grain of sand. The navel or the grain of sand in this metaphor is the Real drive and trauma, which, as a 'hard' given, initiate a process of (layer by layer) meaning-making. It is the opaque root around which the Symbolic-

Imaginary envelope of dreams, symptoms and identity is wrapped. It is a tango between the granular Real and the mother-of-pearl by which this Real is surrounded.

Beneath the subject that emerges and is interpellated by the symbolic order of language and convention and the person with their illusions of imaginary wholeness, there is indeed the insistence of a nameless being. It imposes itself and thus disrupts any form of coherence or closure. It bubbles up from the galvanising directives of drive and trauma. These compel us to an *absolutely different* character beyond any societal norm or convention. After all, we differ from each other primarily in our very own way of dealing with pain/pleasure.

12 *Enjoy your Symptom!* A Lacanian Paradox

In Lacanian psychoanalysis, you can turn necessity into a virtue. Compare it to a poacher becoming a gamekeeper so that the original song gets an entirely different arrangement. Like Nietzsche's *amor fati*, you embrace your (unconscious) fate, or at least the drive or the 'basic fantasy' underlying it. In this way, you can succeed in the call of (the Elvis of psychoanalysis) Slavoj Žižek to 'Enjoy your symptom!'. You then identify with a core of enjoyment that is different for everyone or elsewhere. It lies hidden in the motto: to each their own thing. In Lacan's view, what ultimately drives us is as unique and non-sensical as a fingerprint. You reach the pinnacle of your psychoanalytic process (in a one-liner) by producing your specific exception. Not in a striving for exceptionality but simply by following far enough the idiosyncratic course of your drives and desires.

The reader immediately understands that Jacques Lacan's ideas refer to a form of psychoanalysis that must be distinguished from psychotherapy and other post-Freudians. Getting better is a desirable side effect, primarily aimed at becoming more yourself and, in that sense, absolutely different from everyone else – not in the form of narcissistic distinctiveness but, on the contrary, through a position beyond the mirror.

Throughout his thinking, Lacan, therefore, discusses castration (not to be confused with a veterinary procedure) in its multiple forms. We are alienated from ourselves by the imaginary, divided by symbolic language, and we exhibit the tics of the Real of drive and trauma that continue to insist. Lacanian psychoanalysis recognises our 'castration' as our particular form of imperfection, deficiency and lack. It simultaneously underlies a desire to overcome it. Even against the rain and better judgement!

13 Attachment and Mentalisation

Based on the main inspirations, I have outlined the background of assumptions or pretensions regarding a psychoanalytically understood psychotherapeutic process. To complete this, I would like to add some developments from recent decades. They add many new accents to practice and theory. I will first place them in a historical perspective.

Towards the end of the last century, psychoanalysis threatened to lose its connection with the social and scientific world. From a former leading player in psychiatry, it had become marginalised, if not ridiculed. It retained a leading status only within the philosophical, cultural and human sciences. The fact that it is once again seeking more inspiration from the natural sciences seems to have reversed this decline in recent decades.

To begin with, I would explicitly like to mention the Hungarian-born British psychoanalyst Peter Fonagy for two reasons. Thanks to him, attachment, in conjunction with mentalising capacity, has received growing attention in the psychotherapeutic world. Especially with patients with a history of severe emotional deficits, abuse and trauma, they are decisive factors, both causally and therapeutically.

Every psychotherapy involves relationship and interpretation, but the relative weight of their therapeutic effectiveness differs. Even with the best therapeutic relationship, nothing changes about the neurosis, for example, while in earlier or deeper disorders, it can already be healing and beneficial in itself.

In the line of Charles Darwin (whose intellectual biography he wrote), the British psychoanalyst John Bowlby had already theorised the importance of a secure base/attachment. Fonagy and his colleagues have since shown that the quality of this attachment calibrates both our emotional and physical resilience. Attachment is closely linked to our ability to read our personal and others' mental states. This so-called mentalising capacity allows us to interpret and (re)act to them appropriately so that their impact is tempered.

Depending on the security of our attachment and our capacity for mentalisation, drive and emotion regulation increase, all kinds of blind and evacuative fuss (to 'get rid of it') decreases, and our overall psychosocial stability benefits. They are part of the non-specific therapeutic factors. More specifically, however, psychoanalytically interpretation/awareness must also be added to the beneficial effects of all this.

14 The Scientific Basis: Neuropsychoanalysis

Psychoanalysis had retreated into the seclusion of the consulting room and sought inspiration almost exclusively from within its ranks. Nobel laureate Eric Kandel reproaches it for having long and haughtily failed to legitimise itself according to classical scientific empirical research. Nevertheless, he considers it the most suitable intellectual framework for psychiatry.

Fonagy is also an international advocate in this area. On the one hand, he mobilised a real catch-up effort regarding effectiveness research. Furthermore, concerning psychoanalytic assumptions, he sought connections with cognitive science, attachment research, ethological, primatological and infant research, and the burgeoning neurosciences (boosted, among other things, by high-tech medical imaging). These visualise the essentially invisible and immaterial world of the mental and often contribute to the testing of previous psychoanalytic findings.

On the initiative of the South African neuropsychologist and (later) psychoanalyst Mark Solms, a veritable new discipline emerged since the turn of the millennium: neuropsychoanalysis. It builds on the early (and, as is often forgotten, purely neuro- and natural sciences) Freud. It has already made several innovative contributions. For example, it distinguishes explicit, biographical and declarative memory circuits from implicit and procedural circuits. The former can be told. The latter initially only manifest themselves in patterns of (inter) action. They can, however, be made conscious and explicit in psychotherapy.

While Freud still considered the cerebral cortex the seat of our consciousness, it now appears that the perceptual or cognitive rather than the emotional or instinctual processes are unconscious. Our consciousness is not rooted in the neocortex but in older and deeper brain structures. We are aware of our sexual or aggressive drives or, more broadly, our feelings, but they are often disembodied. They are not (through repression and other defence mechanisms) 'incorrectly' symbolised, that is to say (through processes of displacement and condensation) bound to representations other than the original ones.

Even before Freud, the dream was a *via regia* ('royal road') to the unconscious. It is the guardian of sleep and fulfils wishes in a disguised way. The discovery of paradoxical or REM (rapid eye movement) sleep initially seemed to refute this basic psychoanalytic assumption. The dream was relegated to a physiological phenomenon that we share with animals. Its 'content' was supposedly no more than meaningless noise. However, Solms demonstrated that the dream correlates with but cannot be reduced to paradoxical sleep. In terms of content and in a hallucinatory way, it is indeed marked by wish fulfilment or need satisfaction.

Because Solms has edited a new *Standard Edition* of Freud's complete neurological and psychoanalytic work, he is rapidly becoming one of the most influential psychoanalytic figures. Will he succeed in restoring the scientific prestige of a vilified psychoanalysis? Neuropsychoanalysis can confirm certain Freudian assumptions (for example, concerning transference and resistance) but also falsify others (for example, the id is not unconscious but conscious). As is known, falsifiability is, for the philosopher of science Karl Popper, a necessary condition to even speak of psychoanalysis as a science …

15 Conclusion: Check!

I return to the clinical situation to conclude. The different views on the psychotherapeutic process discussed above do not exclude each other. Depending on the patient or the moment, they are all more, or less, applicable or valid. It is important to remember that all the figures mentioned worked with different types of patients in various settings and within their macro- and micro-culture. In other words, much (so-called) contradiction also has to do with their context and history.

Freud compared the psychoanalytic process to a game of chess. Only the beginning and the end can be formulated more generally. Since each patient and each psychotherapist are unique, each middle-game of the psychotherapeutic process will proceed differently. It is not 'one size fits all', but, as the Australian psychoanalyst Neville Symington says, a constant adaptation and attunement to the evolving idiosyncrasies of the individual.

With the help of our specifically human neocortex, mind-wandering, language, thought and judgement, we try to increase our grasp of and understanding of deeper mental domains. Sooner or later, however, we must acknowledge that we are not (entirely) masters in our own house. Our unconscious leads its own life and household based on pleasure and unpleasure and it occasionally escapes purely rational action. The result is (borrowed from the Flemish modernist poet Paul Van Ostaijen) a '*spleen pour rire*': a melancholy in laughter.

According to the British moralist Horace Walpole, the world is a tragedy to those who feel and a comedy to those who think. By racking your brain and squeezing your soul, you develop a kind of Janus face that allows you to look in two directions. You can think and feel simultaneously but also look both inwards and outwards, to the past and the future, to dreams and reality, to the other and yourself. Stereotypy gives way to stereoscopy. The world gains a new dimension.

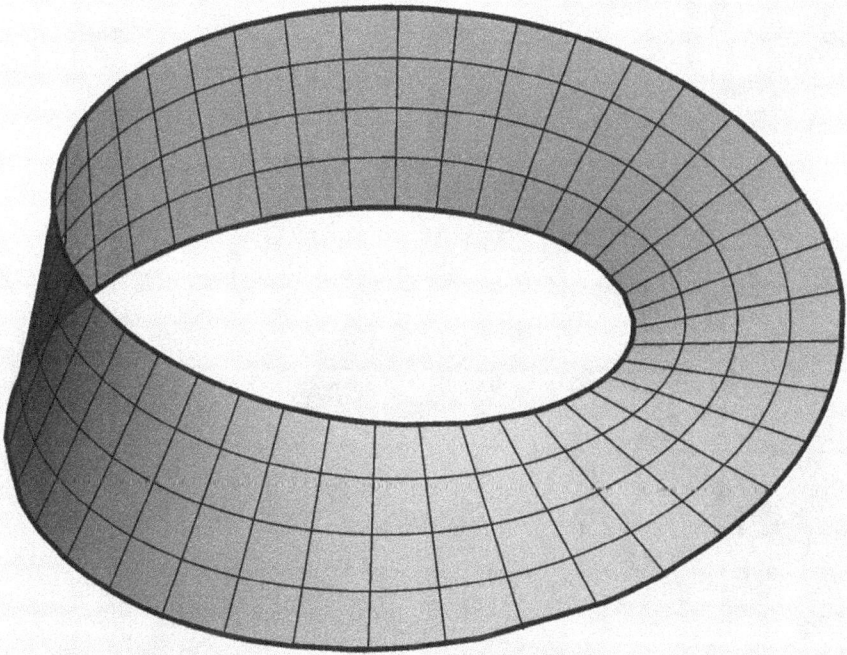

Figure 4.1 Mobius band.

I end with one of Jacques Lacan's famous figures that illustrates this last point: the Mobius band. If you slide your finger along this strip, you imperceptibly end up on the other side. This movement makes palpable how relative the contradictions above are and how the psychotherapeutic journey paradoxically changes nothing and everything simultaneously. One of the patients also explicitly stated this somewhere. Suppose you remember who, my congratulations! You are a close reader.

Chapter 5

Postlude

A Game of Chess

As if caught in a fist
We sit together in the heat
And the street where we
So slowly play seems to
Fit.

You send out a Knight? My
Bishop whispers. His lips are
In sync. So is the wind, holding
Its breath before every
Sigh.

Then there's this lonesome
Fly on your wrist and one trouser
Leg seems too long for the
Other: arousal is surrounding the
Board.

Drops of sweat are skiing down-
Hill: a warning for my
Nostrils to ward off some
Avalanche.

After all, the game isn't
Aimed at thrills but at
Stills.

Mark Kinet

DOI: 10.4324/9781003528067-5

Modus Operandi

As I stated in my stage setting, this book answers a gap. Indeed, it is rare to hear from patients who have gone through psychotherapy and are able or willing to testify about it. In early 2021, I sent the following letter to people whose email addresses I had at my disposal, with whom I was still in contact or who had stopped their treatment with me not too long before.

* * *

L.S.,

In the Psychoanalytisch Actueel *series, I am preparing a thirtieth book. I am asking seventy patients to reflect on their psychotherapeutic process and write a truthful text of approximately 2,500 words. It is essential to reflect on their views for both scientific and societal reasons. Publication will be under your own or fictitious initials. I will take care of some final linguistic editing.*

Herewith are some guiding questions purely for inspiration. What difficulties led me to therapy? What help did I have beforehand? What were my complaints, symptoms, problems? What were my expectations? How did I experience the psychotherapist? How did I experience the psychotherapy? What helped? What did not help? How long did my psychotherapy process take, and why? In what format (inpatient, day therapy, outpatient) and why? What has changed? What did it teach me? Overall, how do I look back on my evolution?

I will provide the book with an extensive introductory preface and a concluding afterword. The submission deadline is 30 April 2021. However, please send your reply by 28 February 2021. I am available via email for any additional questions.
Best regards,
Dr Kinet

* * *

I received thirty-six positive responses on 28 February, of which five of them, for various personal reasons, still gave up before the submission deadline. The ratio of men to women was about fifty-fifty. All kinds of psychiatric and psychological problems were covered.

Following this English adaptation and translation, I emailed 10 other patients the same email in early 2024, asking them to write about their

DOI: 10.4324/9781003528067-6

psychotherapeutic process. Seven responded to this request, including one man and six women.

Altogether, then, this book contains thirty-eight testimonies. Women are slightly in the majority. This is a striking reflection of reality because women are overrepresented in psychiatric settings, while men are overrepresented in detention centres. It is well known that they may struggle with similar issues that manifest themselves differently.

For Product Safety Concerns and Information please contact our EU
representative GPSR@taylorandfrancis.com
Taylor & Francis Verlag GmbH, Kaufingerstraße 24, 80331 München, Germany